NURSING RESEARCH

Carol T. Bush, R.N., Ph.D.

Reston Publishing Company, Inc.
A Prentice-Hall Company
Reston, Virginia

Library of Congress Cataloging in Publication Data

Bush, Carol T.
  Nursing research.

  Bibliography: p.
  1. Nursing—Research. 2. Nursing—Research—
Methodology. I. Title. [DNLM: 1. Nursing.
2. Research—methods. WY 20.5 B978n]
RT81.5.B87 1985   610.73'07'2   84-17863
ISBN 0-8359-5046-8

This book is dedicated to
Aubrey, Keith, Lynnette, and Deirdre
with love.

CONTENTS

Chapter 4.   What are you going to look for?

IDENTIFICATION OF THE VARIABLES   43

Chapter 5.   How do you plan to do it?

RESEARCH DESIGNS   55

Chapter 6.   How do you stick to your plan in the real world?

RESEARCH PROCEDURE AND METHODS   75

Chapter 7.   What are you going to do with it when you get it?

ORGANIZATION AND ANALYSIS OF DATA   89

Chapter 8.   What sense are you going to make of it?

FINDINGS, INTERPRETATIONS, AND
    RECOMMENDATIONS   123

PART II   WRITING THE RESEARCH REPORT   153

Chapter 9.   How are you going to tell others about it?

WRITING THE REPORT AND PUBLISHING   155

PREFACE

This research textbook is designed for undergraduate nursing students. The book is the result of many years of research involvement with graduate and undergraduate students, both in the classroom and as research adviser. My goal has always been, as it is for this volume, to stimulate the interest of students in research by demystifying the research process and demonstrating the relevance of nursing research to nursing practice.

The organization of this book is designed to be a step-by-step guide to doing research. I believe that any nurse can do research and all nurses should have knowledge of research and be able to intelligently apply research findings to practice. Many educators caution that it is unrealistic to expect nurses to conduct independent research projects before the master's (if not the doctoral) level. The point is well taken; no one should ever believe that he or she is a polished researcher without appropriate credentials and extensive experience. Everyone has to start somewhere. I believe the beginning nurse should be exposed to the research process so that the basis for a body of nursing knowledge and sound nursing practice can be understood. The degree of application of the research process will depend on the practice environment, the abilities and interests of the individual nurse, and the educational experiences available.

My experiences with master's degree students have shown me that if they haven't participated in research until the graduate level, many of them literally panic (become unable to function and require crisis intervention) when confronted with the assignment to prepare a thesis proposal. I believe, therefore, in the introduction of research activities at the undergraduate level where the process can be demystified before the students learn to dread it so severely.

ACKNOWLEDGMENTS

Just as a research project develops over a period of time, with input and influence from many individuals and resources, so this book has evolved. I am sincerely grateful to colleagues, teachers, and students for the ways they have molded my attitudes and experiences related to research and writing.

Specifically, the following colleagues have shared research knowledge which is reflected in this book: Dr. Gene Cranston Anderson, Dr. Shirley Carey, Dr. Mary deChesnay, Dr. Sylvia Fields, Dr. LaRetta Garland, Dr. Maggie Gilead, Dr. Josephine Jones, Dr. Jean Megenity, Ms. Pamela Moore, Dr. Leah Gorman, Dr. Rose McGee, Dr. Jane Mulaik, Dr. Marcene Powell, and Dr. Elizabeth Sharp. I am very grateful for their support.

Graduates from the master's of nursing program kindly consented to allow excerpts from their works to be included and critiqued. Special thanks is extended to: Barbara Anderson, Debbie Gunter, Karen Baer Himmelstein, Brenda Knaack, Audrey Nelson, Debbie Nichols, and Joanna Wright.

I am sincerely grateful to Dr. Sharol F. Jacobson, Director of Nursing Research at the University of Oklahoma, for her repeated reviews of manuscripts of the text. Dr. Jacobson's comments always included exquisite recommendations and, even more importantly, encouragement.

I am grateful to the Literary Executor of the late Sir Ronald A. Fisher, F.R.S., to Dr. Frank Yates, F.R.S., and to Longman Group, Ltd., London, for permission to reprint Tables IV and VII from their book *Statistical Tables for Biological, Agricultural and Medical Research* (6th Edition, 1974).

INTRODUCTION

The goal of this text is to demystify the research process so that all nurses may become comfortable with and challenged by the rewards (and frustrations) of research activities and reports. In order to accomplish this goal, the book is divided into five parts. Part I is the research process and contains eight chapters that include the identification of a researchable problem, how to review the literature and what to get from it, utilizing conceptual frameworks, definition and measurement of variables, recognition and selection of research designs, employment of research procedure and methods, organization and analysis of data, and generalization and application of findings. Part II contains one chapter that includes guidelines for writing a research report—what to include and how it should be presented. Part III presents guidelines for critiquing a research report. Whether one should be able to critique research before doing it or if doing it helps one know what to look for is an unresolved debate. The approach taken in this book is that doing research is not only possible but fun, and after one has gotten one's feet wet, one then has a basis for criticizing the research products of others. Therefore, the book covers the entire research process, from experiencing a problem to writing a report, before dealing with issues of critique, ethics, and why nurses should do research. Parts IV and V cover the latter two topics.

The purposes of this text are to
- Guide the beginning researcher through the research process
- Facilitate the critical reading of nursing and related research
- Stimulate the intelligent application of research findings to clinical practice
- Stimulate nurses' awareness of the myriad researchable and research-needed questions encountered in daily practice

and to guide the beginning researcher through the research process.

PART I
THE RESEARCH PROCESS

The first part of this book contains a discussion of the research process. Research begins with a *motivation* (either *internal,* as wanting to answer a clinical question, or *external,* as wanting to obtain a degree which requires a thesis or research project). The process includes: identification of the research question (Chapter 1); review of the literature (Chapter 2) and formulation of conceptual frameworks (Chapter 3); identification and measurement of variables (Chapter 4); research designs (Chapter 5); procedure and research methods (Chapter 6); organization and statistical treatment of data (Chapter 7); and presentation of findings with recommendations for nursing practice and further research (Chapter 8).

The purpose of Part I is to provide a guide for the beginning researcher to become aware of the myriad of researchable and research-needed questions encountered in the daily activities of nursing. As awareness increases, the nurse will begin to formulate questions and seek answers through systematic investigation.

Chapter 1

What have you been wondering about as you practice nursing?

IDENTIFYING RESEARCH QUESTIONS

Chapter Objectives

Upon successful completion of this chapter, the student will be able to

- Differentiate the research process from other approaches to problems
- Identify potentially researchable problems from the experiences of the student
- Name three sources of research questions
- Formulate research questions from problems identified
- Understand the circuitous direction characteristic of the research process

INTRODUCTION

You probably did not decide to be a nurse in order to conduct research. Let's be honest—you probably did not elect to take this course or read this book eagerly or voluntarily. However, since you are here and you are reading the book—at least this far—why not make the most of the situation and get out of it all you possibly can?

Think back to something you do like and that is meaningful to you. Assuming that you find satisfaction working with your clients in the clinical setting, what happened the last time you were there? Did anyone—nursing assistant, nurse, physician—say or do anything that you questioned, felt uncomfortable with, or that surprised you? Did any client have discomfort, physical or emotional, that you did not seem to be able to relieve and no one else could either? Did it appear that anyone was doing something (writing on the client's record, counting narcotics, making out schedules, ordering supplies, taking specimens to the laboratory) when you thought that there was a need for help elsewhere (a client was crying, you had some questions that went unanswered, one of the staff nurses seemed to be harassed in trying to provide care for each of her clients)? Did a client complain about the care she was receiving? Did you overhear any comments about staff staying out sick more than seemed reasonable? Did the physicians complain about the nurses or the nurses complain about the physicians or the aides? In the community agency, are mothers complaining about the high cost of food and the difficulty they have providing nutritional meals on a limited budget? How would you attempt to find answers or solutions to any of these or innumerable other questions or problems that arise in any clinical setting?

You've got it! You could do some research. Of course there are other ways to solve problems and seek answers to questions.

APPROACHES TO PROBLEMS

Ignore or Redefine Problems

You can ignore the problems or define them as belonging to someone else. If nurses are abusing sick leave, it is not your problem—or is it? What about the client you dreamed about—not your responsibility; but whose job is it to investigate ways of making that client, and the others similar to him, more comfortable? Sure, you are only a student or a staff nurse or just beginning to think about what this thing called research is all about. Think about it. Someone really should do it, and that someone might as well be you. Or, if you don't do it, who will? And when?

Trial and Error

If you chose not to disown the problem, you might attempt a trial-and-error approach; that is, do something and see if it works. If it does, do it again. If it doesn't, try something else. Of course, in the clinical setting you exercise professional judgment and responsibility in whatever you do. The criticism of the trial-and-error approach is that it is not efficient and, in fact, may be inappropriate.

Tradition or Authority

Oh, how many procedures nurses follow because "that's the way we've always done it." Some of those procedures will stand the test of scientific inquiry, but research is needed to determine what should be retained, modified, and replaced. Some authority, too, is appropriate particularly as related to standards formulated by such recognized bodies as the American Nurses' Association. Florence Nightingale, as a nursing authority, had some profound ideas, such as the beneficial effects of hygiene and fresh air (Nightingale 1969). Legal authority seems unchallengeable, but with research evidence, laws can be changed; nurse practice acts are continually undergoing revisions.

Problem Solving and Nursing Process

Another way to seek answers and solve problems is to use the problem-solving approach. First, you identify the problem. Name it. Define it. Think about it and make sure that you know exactly what it is you want to solve. Second, gather information about the problem. When does it occur? What is happening at the time of the occurrence of the problem? Who always seems to be involved? Third, think about all of the things you might do to solve the problem—from nothing to absurdity. Brainstorm. Be creative. Make up funny solutions—and laugh. Fourth, systematically take each of the viable solutions you have thought of and think through what would happen if you implemented that particular one. It helps to write down the possible solutions and the probable outcomes. Fifth, considering the outcomes, choose the solution that seems best and try it. Sixth, evaluate the results. Did it work? What was successful and what failed? If it worked, what are you going to tackle next? If it did not work, try another solution until one works or go back to the first step in problem solving.

No doubt, this is not your first exposure to the problem-solving approach. If this makes sense to you and you have some success in using it, why should you consider research? How does research differ from problem solving? When you have successfully sought and found a solution to a specific problem using the problem-solving approach, you know what worked that time, but you do not necessarily know if it would work again. You also may not have any assurance that the same solution would work in another situation. You have not necessarily *described* the various factors in the situation precisely enough that anyone else could take what you have demonstrated and effectively apply it, even in the same situation; and, even less likely, in another situation. You have not *controlled* all of the elements in the environment to the extent that you can know that what you did really accounts for the results. In addition, you have not necessarily reviewed what has been written about the problem and solutions that have been attempted by others. Therefore, how do your results relate to what has been done or attempted in the past? Actually, someone else may be doing the same thing or something better. In other words, you cannot generalize your results to other situations.

Finally, what principles or concepts are involved in what you have done or discovered? What conceptual framework does the problem fit into? Especially in nursing as a young profession, it is important that we build a body of knowledge that is characteristic of, if not unique to, nursing. As an applied discipline, it is important that we communicate important clinical findings to each other and other disciplines as indicated.

The problem-solving process is familiar to the reader, for it is not unlike the nursing process. The outline below shows the steps in the two processes.

PROBLEM SOLVING	NURSING PROCESS
1. Problem identification	1. Client assessment
2. Information gathering	2. Diagnosis
3. Solutions suggestions	3. Plan
4. Outcome considerations	
5. Solution choice	
6. Solution implementation and evaluation	4. Implementation
	5. Evaluation

Note that the *number* of steps in problem solving and the nursing process differ from one source to another. You may have been taught four or six steps in the nursing process. The number is not as important as the concept of the order of the process. The similarities between problem solving and the nursing process are: the beginning with a concern or problem, the gathering of information (included in the assessment phase of the nursing process), the step of making a decision as to what to do, and the implementation and evaluation of that decision.

The differences begin with the possible source of the concern. With problem solving, the source may be a situation, a procedure, a person, or a policy. The nursing process begins with a client and the nurse; the concern is health related (mental, physical, social, or environmental). The primary source of information is the client (including complaints, history, physical examination, and laboratory tests). A nursing diagnosis is made based on the assessment. In problem solving, the possible solutions and outcomes are the results of a creative process of considering novel ways of dealing with an as-yet-unsolved (at least, for that individual at that time) problem. The nursing diagnosis should provide the nurse with relatively clear directions as to what should be done for the client. In the rigorous situation, nursing protocols will have been established so that the steps to implement are outlined. Of course, each client is unique, and the nurse must adapt any procedure to the individual client. Evaluation of the problem solving, as well as the nursing process, is successful if the expected outcome is produced. If the problem solving evaluation is not favorable, the best solution may not have been implemented; if the nursing process is not successful, the nurse must go back to reconsider the diagnosis, which may necessitate additional data gathering.

The next topic is the research process, which also has parallels with problem solving and the nursing process.

Research and Problem Solving

Recalling that the research process may have any number of steps, depending on how finely you choose to break them down, we will begin by considering the process in nine steps. The first three steps, as identified here (identifying the problem, reviewing the literature, and framing the problem in a theoretical context) are interchangeable. As suggested earlier, clinical practice is a source of research problems; two other sources are nursing literature and theory. That is, instead of pulling from your experiences, you may go to the library and read nursing research journals or books on nursing theories. Either or both of these references are fertile sources of research problems.

After you have proceeded through the first three steps in any order (realistically, you probably go back and forth among the three), you must refine the problem you wish to study by framing it in a research question form or in an hypothesis (much more about hypothesis-generating in Chapter 4). The fifth step of outlining the methodology includes choosing the appropriate research design and specifying *exactly* how you will conduct the research (Chapters 5 and 6). After obtaining all appropriate permissions, you are ready to collect data according to the plan you devised. Analyzing the data is the seventh step in our nine-step system. The eighth step is the interpretation of the data (the findings), with the final step being that of drawing conclusions and making recommendations for practice and further research.

A comparison of the research and the problem-solving processes should help you understand that the research process is characterized by being placed in a context of what has been previously known (other research findings) or presumed (theory). This relationship to the work of others and rigorous adherence to the data collection make it possible to generalize research findings so that they might be meaningful to others in addition to the researcher. Conversely, problem solving is considered to be specific to the situation and individuals involved in a particular problem at a particular time. While problem solving may help you know what to do with the next client who has the same complaint, it is not likely to help others in similar situations.

The following outline contains the research steps and places the problem solving process in parallel for comparison.

RESEARCH	PROBLEM SOLVING
1. Problem identification	1. Problem identification
2. Literature review	2. Information gathering
3. Problem framing in theory	
4. Questions posed or hypothesis generated	3. Solutions suggested
	4. Outcomes considered
5. Methodology outlined	5. Solution chosen
6. Data collected	6. Solution implemented and evaluated
7. Data analyzed	
8. Findings interpreted	
9. Conclusions drawn and recommendations made	

Research can be fun and exciting as well as important. Research need not be overwhelming, unmanageable, dull, or grueling, even though some of us have chosen to make it so. We make such a big thing of "writing the proposal" (steps one through five, plus an indication of how the data will be analyzed) that graduate students become immobilized at the thought of the task. They often have difficulty putting the first word on paper because of the anxiety that has been created by the emphasis and mystique associated with a thesis or dissertation. The revelation that such pain is unnecessary is by no means a license for doing poorly designed or improperly executed research; it simply means that you can start simple, keep it clean, and build until you have useful, generalizable data.

WHAT IS RESEARCHABLE?

Anything that can be described, quantified, or measured is potentially researchable. Obviously "potentially" is a key word here. Getting control of the research variables becomes a challenge. (Variables are simply phenomena of importance in the study—more about variables in Chapter 4). Areas of research interest may be categorized into five foci: (1) nurse characteristics, (2) client characteristics, (3) nursing administration, (4) nursing education, and (5) nursing care of clients.

1. *Nurse characteristics.* You may be interested in nurses. Why do they choose to work in a given specialty area? What gives them the most satisfaction in their jobs? What factors are associated with a high rate of absenteeism?

2. *Client characteristics.* Perhaps you are interested in client variables. What expectations does the client have of the nurses or other health care providers? What variables are associated with postoperative infections? What characteristics of mothers are associated with an increased probability of child abuse?

3. *Nursing administration.* Nursing administration is the focus of many studies and justifiably so, for leadership in nursing is one of the most critical problems nurses face. What variables contribute to successful leadership in a nurse? How are successful nursing leaders prepared for their positions? How do effective nursing leaders enhance nursing practice so that nurses can make a difference in the promotion of health?

4. *Nursing education.* Nursing education is another important focus of research. How does one recruit creative, energetic individuals into nursing? How do you keep students interested and motivated to become dedicated to nursing? What content is important?

5. *Nursing care of clients.* What does the nurse do that contributes to the promotion of health in the clients for whom the nurse is responsible? This is the key question in nursing. The implications are serious. This core question should be the central focus of all nursing research even if some of the studies seem peripheral. Which of two presurgical preparations facilitates earlier hospital discharge? What type of nursing handling of premature infants promotes weight gain? For every study

you read, ask the question: What are the implications for nursing? If this process seems obvious, in reality it is frequently overlooked.

Unresearchable Questions

Regardless of the focus of your research, ethical considerations are of paramount importance. Many questions are useful and interesting but do not lend themselves to investigation because of ethical consideration of how human beings should be treated. For example, you do not plan to separate twins born to a mother diagnosed as schizophrenic in order to study the effects of environment no matter how interesting this information might be. Neither would you withhold medication from a client who is in considerable pain to determine if the client will recover faster if medication is withheld. Sound nursing judgment and ethical consideration of clients are necessary ingredients of all nursing research.

Interdisciplinary Research

Although nursing research focuses on the areas indicated above, the contributions of nonnurses to several of these areas is recognized. One of the reasons nurses have a responsibility to be informed about the research process is so that they can intelligently participate (or decline to participate) in the research being conducted by others. Working with members of other disciplines in conducting research can be stimulating and is being encouraged by nurse researchers and their colleagues as well as by funding agencies.

FROM RESEARCH PROBLEM AREA TO RESEARCH QUESTION

Getting from the research problem area, or some sort of vague feeling of uneasiness, frustration, or concern, to a research question is not always easy. The research problem area has to be narrow to a point that allows the researcher to proceed in a clear direction. Suppose, for example, you notice that residents of a nursing home are markedly unenthusiastic about meal times. They show little interest in what is served, their appetites appear to be depressed, and they grumble about the terrible food they are given. If there is something about this situation you would like to investigate, you have the choice of several research areas: the appetites of all elderly individuals, the appetites of elderly individuals who live in nursing homes, the nutritional condition of the residents of this nursing home, the quality of food in this, or a sampling of, nursing homes, food preferences of elderly individuals, other factors associated with food consumption such as the time of day it is served. This list is virtually endless, but the point is that you have to decide what area you want to focus on.

How do you decide on the focus of your research project? First, you might observe the situation to see what seems to be outstanding about it. Is the serving time unusual such as dinner at 4:30 p.m.? Is the food cold? Simultaneously, you might try checking out your hunch with others who have an opportunity to make similar observations or with the residents themselves. What have they observed? Do their observations fit with yours? Meanwhile, you start reading about anything that relates to the situation: food services in nursing homes; the physiology of taste and how the aging process affects taste; the social symbolism associated with food; the importance of choices of food; food customs and their impact on the practices of elderly individuals.

Now with this additional information from a variety of sources, you are in a position to zero in on what you and probably others are interested in knowing more about. Many students believe that their research must differ markedly from anything that anyone else has ever done or thought about. Not so—do not hesitate to discuss your research ideas with peers, faculty, administrators, or other researchers, for they may be invaluable sources of encouragement and helpful ideas. If you propose a good idea in the clinical area, nursing supervisors will be in a position to help you obtain the necessary permissions to implement your plan. In the school setting, faculty have knowledge of resources that may not be generally known. Faculty can help you think through your ideas and avoid some pitfalls. Conversely, if you discuss your ideas with someone who is less than enthusiastic (unfortunately some individuals can be bitingly critical) do not be discouraged. Remember that the greatest scientists have suffered ridicule. Try to be objective (it's hard when you are hurt) and consider what was instructive about the criticism. Use the appropriate suggestions, read some more about your research area, and talk to someone else.

Once you have identified the specific area of a problem you want to investigate, put it in the form of a question. Lindeman and Schantz (1982) suggested three criteria for a good research question. A good research question

1. Can be answered by collecting observable evidence of empirical data
2. Contains reference to the relationship between two or more variables
3. Follows logically and consistently from what is already known about the topic. (p. 6)

The more specific you can be, the better you will be able to proceed.

Key words in formulating a research question are *specificity, narrowness,* and *relationship.* Specificity refers to the process of clarifying exactly what you want to study—nutritional deficiencies, food habits, adolescents' sexual knowledge, or infant sleeping patterns. While this seems obvious, it is frequently very difficult. You may say, "I'm interested in pregnant women," or you may indicate concerns about alcoholics, or mentally retarded adolescents, or individuals on kidney dialysis. What is it about these individuals that concerns you? Be specific—prevention of ankle edema in pregnant women during the third trimester, providing effective incentives to keep alcoholics in treatment programs, developing sex education programs for moderately mentally retarded adolescents, or providing emotional support for individuals on kidney dialysis. If you are specific about what you want to study, you will be able to communicate your interest to others. If you cannot seem to make others understand what your project is about, you may not have gotten specific enough.

Narrowness is another obvious, but troublesome, concept in asking a research question. If you are going to do a study, you may believe that you should find out all there is to know about the area. Wrong. It is more desirable to be reasonably sure of specific information you uncover about a segment of a problem than to endanger the whole project by biting off more that you can chew. Another problem with global investigations is that the researcher is often overwhelmed with data that are unmanageable if not meaningless. (Don't catch more fish than you are willing to clean.) Narrow the question to a manageable size by considering what you can handle in terms of feasibility of time, money, talent, and staff. Are you really interested in all pregnant women or only those in a high risk clinic? Do you want to know when ankle edema occurs or if support hose will reduce and/or prevent ankle edema in pregnant women during the third trimester? When is the optimum gestation time for the subject to begin wearing support hose? Do you want to study all female alcoholics or adolescent female alcoholics served by a community mental health program? Perhaps your interest could be narrowed to moderately mentally retarded male adolescents in a group living situation. Narrow your research question so that you can manage it.

What is the relationship of the variables you are interested in studying? The research question should be clear about whether you are questioning a cause and effect relationship, asking if two or more variables seem to usually occur together without suggesting cause and effect, or whether you are interested in systematically describing what you observe under certain conditions. A cause and effect relationship is implied in a question such as "Does cigarette smoking predispose individuals to heart disease?" An association without suggesting cause is evident in the question: "Is there a relationship between alcoholism and unemployment?" A descriptive study would be the type that might ask, "What are the play patterns of three-year-old children in day care centers?" Be sure your question is asked appropriately for what you want to know. The more specifically you phrase your question, the tighter you can design your study, and the more dependable your findings will be.

You will find that research does not proceed in a straight line. Once you have formulated the best possible question for your project, you are not safe from having to reconsider at a later point. As you go on to the review of the literature and the selection and application of a conceptual framework, you may need to retreat and reformulate the research question. Your proposal may possibly "drift"; that is, each individual section may be great, but the parts do not hang together as a whole. Keep rechecking the whole for congruence. Be flexible, be willing to reconsider. Your goal is the discovery of new knowledge. Such a serious endeavor must not be compromised because you are unwilling to go back and acknowledge that there might be a better way of phrasing your research question.

FORMULATING THE QUESTION
IS HALF THE BATTLE

In a sense, research reports are deceptive. Reports are presented in a smooth and ordered sequence of thought, action, and analysis. The new researcher soon learns that the actual research process is not so smooth and orderly. An unexpectedly large share of the total time for a research project is spent in formulating the question clearly. Consider Sandra's experiences.

Sandra was a member of a class assigned to complete a research project in order to get credit for the required course. A deadline for identifying a research area of interest was set and rapidly approaching. Sandra was interested in elderly individuals and announced to her class that she wanted to do her study on the older adults in the suburb where she was having clinical experiences. Her faculty adviser agreed that research related to older adults is needed. It is, indeed, an area in which nursing has a grand opportunity to make valuable contributions.

When the adviser asked for Sandra to be more specific about what she wanted to study, Sandra identified health as the area of concern. Health of elderly individuals was still much too broad for Sandra to investigate. Sandra had a strong commitment to the elderly individuals with whom she was working. She felt that their health was threatened by inadequate care. Sandra had observed that when her clients complained to the primary caregivers, their complaints were not taken seriously. Instead, the clients were dismissed as being "senile" or "cranky." Sandra reported that the clients were treated in a condescending manner and symptoms were dismissed as "just old age." Sandra believed that medications were prescribed to placate the clients, resulting in drowsy, lethargic, compliant individuals.

It was clear that Sandra had made some observations that had caused her concern. The concern was legitimate. The observations and inferences may have been accurate. Sandra was very clear that she wanted to study health in older adults, and she perceived the adviser as dense or inflexible as the adviser attempted to lead Sandra to a specific, narrow question with clearly identified relationships. The adviser tried not to dictate what Sandra should study or do the study for her. Sandra felt threatened and her defense was to abandon the topic. Again, the adviser assured Sandra that research related to health and elderly individuals was appropriate and needed; she urged Sandra to retain the topic, go to the library, and read recent studies that were related to Sandra's interest.

Although initially Sandra was bewildered by the conglomeration of literature on the health care of elderly individuals, she began to notice something very interesting. No differentiation was made among subgroups of the population. Everyone over the age of 65 seemed to be lumped together as though they all had the same needs and resources. Males, females, black, white, rural, urban were treated as though they were all alike. Sandra's interest intensified for she had observed that the clients in the rural area where she was practicing were having difficulty getting adequate transportation to health care facilities. Clients in the city had public transportation available for travel to health centers.

Sandra formulated the following research question: Are there differences in the adequacy and availability of health care as perceived by individuals over 65 years of age according to sex, race, or geographic location? Sex obviously referred to males and females; Sandra defined race as black or white according to the category on the questionnaire checked by the subject; and geographic location was divided into rural and urban according to the location of the health center serving the client.

The struggle by both Sandra and her adviser seemed long and difficult from the point of Sandra's indication of interest in knowing more about elderly individuals to the formulation of a research question with clear definitions of the key terms. The struggle was rewarding, for Sandra conducted a study that both interested her and provided useful information.

SUMMARY

Research is a part of real life. The questions must relate to something meaningful that you identify from your experiences, the literature, or theory. Questions may be associated with clinical practice, characteristics of nurses or clients, nursing administration, or nursing education; the ultimate goal being to demonstrate that nursing care promotes health in individuals, groups, families, and communities. From your initial hunch, you will make further observations, talk the problem over with others who are knowledgeable about the situation, and check the literature for what others are doing about the problem. Refine your research question by paying particular attention to specificity, narrowness, and relationships.

The following suggestions and exercises are intended to help you experience the process described so far. Chapter 2 includes a discussion of systematic review of relevant literature.

Suggestions for Further Study

There is no substitute for practice if one is to develop as a researcher. The following exercises may be done by individuals, but they will be far more instructive if used as class experiences.

1. Identify something from your recent experiences that you would like to investigate and follow it through with the steps presented so far.
   a) What is your hunch, concern, problem?
   b) What do others think? Have they been aware of the problem? Do they see it differently from the way you do?
   c) What has been written about this problem recently? Is the popular approach consistent with your observations? What are you asking that is different?
   d) What do you observe about that problem as you consider it further? When does it occur? Who is involved when it occurs? Does it happen every time or only sometimes? Describe the problem objectively.
   e) Formulate the problem into a researchable question.
2. Share your research question with your peers. Discuss the questions you have formulated as to their specificity, narrowness, and clarity of relationships.

3. Select research questions from current nursing and other research journals. Discuss the selections as you did your own research question. How do they compare?

Suggestions for Additional Reading

Abdellah, F. G., and Levine, E. *Better Patient Care through Nursing Research* (2nd edition). New York: Macmillan Publishing Company, Inc., 1979. (Chapters 3 and 5)

Eells, M. A. W. "The Research Problem," in S.D. Krampitz and N. Pavlovich (Eds.), *Readings for Nursing Research.* St. Louis: The C. V. Mosby Company, 1981.

Fox, D. J. *Fundamentals of Research in Nursing* (4th edition). Norwalk, CN: Appleton-Century-Crofts, 1982. (Chapters 2 and 3)

Fuller, E. O. "Selecting a Clinical Nursing Problem for Research," *Image,* 1982, *14*(2), pp. 60–61.

Lindeman, C. A., and Schantz, D. "The Research Question," *The Journal of Nursing Administration,* 1982, January, pp. 6–10.

Polit, D. F., and Hungler, B. P. *Nursing Research: Principles and Methods* (2nd edition). Philadelphia: J. B. Lippincott Company, 1983. (Chapters 2 and 3)

Seaman, C. C., and Verhonick, P. J. *Research Methods for Undergraduate Students in Nursing* (2nd edition). New York: Appleton-Century-Crofts, 1982. (Chapter 3)

Chapter 2
What have others done about it?

REVIEW OF THE LITERATURE

Chapter Objectives

Upon successful completion of this chapter, the student will be able to

- Obtain relevant literary resources pertinent to a topic of inquiry
- Choose systematically the resources relevant to the topic
- Obtain from the resources the information needed for documenting and justifying research on the topic

INTRODUCTION

Once you have some idea of what you want to investigate, the next concern might be "What have others done about this problem"? Others may have thought about it, observed it, or conducted sophisticated experiments related to it. The library is obviously the first source to consider in uncovering this information. At the same time think about what it all means. How does your problem fit with concepts you are familiar with or theories you have learned? What is the concept that is most pertinent to the identified problem? Searches for related research and for a conceptual framework may be done sequentially or simultaneously. As noted in Chapter 1, the research question may come from either the review of the literature or the conceptual framework. Chapter 2 provides suggestions for reviewing the literature while Chapter 3 explains theories, conceptual frameworks, and models.

WHAT TO REVIEW AND HOW

You have decided that you want to study alcoholism among students in public high schools. Where do you begin in the library? Although you may be encouraged by faculty and librarians to start with a computer search of your topic, many nurse researchers believe very strongly that a "hands-on plunge into the literature" should precede computer search. This author agrees; by familiarizing yourself with the card catalog entries related to your topic and by using available abstracts and going to the stacks, you will have a better sense of the context of your topic and will be able to discover the key words necessary to do a successful computer search when the time comes. Unstructured computer searches are not only expensive, they are cluttered with sources that are not even in the ballpark.

After you are comfortable with and conversant about your topic, approach the librarian who will inform you of the cost of running a computer search on your topic. You will get lists of references from any sources you choose depending on the nature of the search conducted. Annotated bibliographies are available and most helpful in determining which entries will be relevant to your study. Computer searches range from a general search of the literature to searches limited to literature from specified disciplines or during limited time periods.

Given that you begin as suggested by doing the initial literature search yourself, the order in which you approach the resources is not critical. You may start with the topic or with names of prominent investigators. Author searches are often more fruitful than subject searches. The point is that by browsing around the library you serendipitously encounter resources that the computer would not have identified simply because you had not crystallized your thoughts well enough to feed the appropriate data into the computer.

Look at the latest issues of journals most likely to contain articles of interest to your project. There are a couple of reasons for this approach: first, these references will not have been made available in computerized indices yet, and, second, they might be more up to date than books because of the usual time lag in getting volumes into print (although the lag in journals is quite lengthy in some cases). If you are fortunate enough to find related articles, there is much to be learned from them. Of course, there is the information relevant to your topic, but there is much more. The reference list is perhaps the most valuable part of the article. From there you can follow those resources of interest. Note that certain references and certain authors will repeatedly appear. Obviously, these are the important ones—read them.

Another approach, which is valuable for topics that have not been researched extensively, is the historical one. Find through the card index, or other indices or computer searches, the first work to appear in the literature. Follow through until the work became diverse and at that point you must make a decision to narrow your scope or perhaps to lengthen the estimated time of your project. (Lengthening your days is not advised—many have attempted it but to no avail.) You will discover that a certain author or group, or center, seems to address best the problem you are investigating. Go with that lead, but do not let blinders keep you from picking up on newcomers who might surface.

A word of advice before you go another step: KEEP ADEQUATE NOTES. Many a person has sadly, reluctantly, not to mention angrily, dragged back to the library to resurrect some obscure volume because an adviser has indicated that the notation or description of the entry is insufficient. The researcher often finds the source has been lost, stolen, or the page ripped out. Many advisers advocate the use of index cards with such fervor that it seems heretical to enter a library without a stack of five-by-seven's. Frankly, index cards seem unhandy. They fall out of notebooks; they are rarely large enough to record what you need; and if you use two cards for the same reference, you cannot find both cards at the same time. Try a loose leaf notebook so that you can record all you need on as many pages as necessary, secure them in the notebook, rearrange them as indicated, and be efficient.

What you need to record varies with your purpose, obviously. As a suggestion, however, the following guide has been useful for reviewing research articles.

1. *A description of the subjects.* Many sweeping conclusions based on a limited number of subjects or a biased sample have appeared in the literature. Who were the subjects? Were they a sample drawn from across the country, in New York City only, across the southeast, or in rural areas? Were the subjects representative of various ethnic groups? How old were they? Was the number evenly distributed across the age range involved? Were both sexes represented, and if so, were they represented evenly? Most of all, how many subjects were there? Although it is not necessarily true that the better study is the one that has the most subjects, you should remain skeptical of generalizations made from studies with a limited number of circumscribed subjects.

2. *How were the data collected?* What research approach was used? What was the research design? What tools were used? Was it a questionnaire, an interview form, or a mailed checklist? Who collected the data—experienced researchers or clinicians whose primary objective was treating the subject for some health-related complaint? Were the tools well-known from having been used in other research? Was the tool developed for this project? Was it tested for validity and reliability? If so, was it tested on a population that had characteristics similar to the one reported? In general, a tool pretested on children undergoing heart surgery may not be valid for children scheduled for tonsillectomies. If the tool used was one that is well-established, was it administered according to the standard procedures?

3. *What are the findings?* This question is important because researchers might have a tendency to get overly enthusiastic about their investigations and skip over the findings to draw conclusions that support their hunches. Always read research with a questioning attitude. What did the research actually find? Six out of eleven may be a majority, but do you want to invest your efforts on data that are not more outstanding than that? On the other hand, if the study was on the benefits of some life-preserving device which resulted in the survival of six individuals when the previous survival rate had been zero, six out of eleven is impressive. Look at the findings literally—what are the figures? What did the researcher actually discover? Examine the figures and tables. What do they communicate?

4. *What are the conclusions drawn by the investigator?* Note that these are the investigator's conclusions and report them as such. Be very careful to record and report the conclusions just as the investigator did. Whether the investigator reported that 15-year-olds have low self-esteem or that a given percentage of pregnant 15-year-olds have self-esteem scores

that are lower than the previously established norm for 15-year-olds is important. To report that mothers responded positively to prenatal classes is not as meaningful as to conclude that prenatal classes reduce the incidence of child abuse.

5. *Do the conclusions drawn make sense to you?* Just because an article is in a reputable journal does not mean that it is irrefutable. Quite the contrary—good research reporting gives you enough detail so that you can intelligently question the results or conclusions; or so that you could replicate the study, which means to repeat it exactly as the original one was done, to determine if the same results will be obtained. If the conclusions do not make sense to you, ask someone else to help you understand it. If it turns out that informed individuals have questions similar to yours, write to the author for clarification. If you disagree, after appropriate consultation with experienced researchers, a letter to the editor of the journal is in order. Research is fun—it's like a game in which an investigator tries to produce as tight a study as possible and test it on peers. The researcher must develop an attitude of acceptance of criticism, for if anything receives any attention, it is most likely to receive criticism.

As you search the literature, read questioningly, carefully, and critically. *How* you review is just as important as *what* you review. All of this reviewing takes much time and concentration. It is better, and in the long run more efficient, to gather more information than you need than to have to go back and retrieve something that you did not adequately review. (Don't forget that copying machines are available in most libraries and, depending on your money-to-time ratio, you may want to use them liberally.)

Usually if you get to this point and you are bored, something is wrong. Either you are bogged down in some trivia that may not be entirely relevant to your research topic, or you chose the wrong topic. Most investigators begin to feel a sense of excitement and discovery as they uncover new truths in print. You may be led to some divergent path and change your focus—that's fine. Go with your interest and momentum within the constraints under which you are working—time, money, advisement.

You should also be aware that research gets easier with experience. After several related studies, you will have a literature reservoir and research process that fit your interests. You will have identified and internalized a theory (or combination of theories) from which you will generate your research questions. Others will begin to notice what you are producing and ask questions. You will have become an expert.

In order to illustrate the content that should be included in a review of the literature, the following excerpt is included. This review was chosen because it includes several important features: selection of relevant literature from an enormous pool; integration of literature from several content areas; an introduction to the review to inform the reader of what is to be covered; subheadings to organize the text; and a summary of the works reviewed with discussion of how the study will relate to what has been done previously. The research question to which this literature review was directed was: Will overweight individuals who have internal locus of control be more successful in losing weight as a result of participation in a weight reduction group than overweight individuals who have external locus of control? [Comments throughout the excerpt will appear in brackets.]

EXCERPT 2-1 _____

LOCUS OF CONTROL AND SUCCESSFUL WEIGHT LOSS
REVIEW OF THE LITERATURE

A review of the literature pertinent to the study included an overview of writings related to the constructs of locus of control and weight loss. In the first area, locus of control (LOC) and weight loss were reviewed. In the second area, an overview of research demonstrating changes in locus of control are presented.

[*The researcher has outlined the areas of literature she covered in the review. Note that this first paragraph informs the reader of what to expect in the review of the literature and how it will be arranged. This feature is both desirable and usually required for theses and dissertations: "Tell the readers what it is you are going to tell them." Following this introductory paragraph is a subheading to acknowledge the beginning of the literature on that topic.*]

LOCUS OF CONTROL RELATED TO WEIGHT LOSS

O'Bryan (1972) studied 54 women participating in a Take Off Pounds Safely (TOPS) weight reduction program. Using a descriptive design, he measured internal-external (I-E) orientation of subjects. O'Bryan was interested in how overweight individuals would score as a group on the internal-external dimension and how those who scored high internal or high external would perform in information seeking, learning, and use of relevant weight-control information. The overweight individuals were found to be significantly more external in orientation. Members of the external group were less likely to report successful experience in weight loss and more likely to attribute their weight problem to physiological causes. Contrary to expectations, no significant differences were found between the internal and external groups on willingness to pursue behavioral materials that might be useful in their own weight reduction programs. Although the volunteer sampling procedure limited the control of extraneous variables, the finding of increased externality in the obese population is supported in the literature.

[*Notice that the researcher reported the method and design of the study reviewed. In addition, she critiqued the study; that is, she noted limitations in the study: ". . . volunteer sampling procedure limited the control of extraneous variables." The findings in the study reviewed was put in the broader context of other literature: ". . . the finding of increased externality in the obese population is supported in the literature." In the study reviewed below, the researcher includes the number of subjects in the sample.*]

Wallston, Wallston, Kaplan, and Maides (1976) studied 34 overweight women to test the hypothesis that subjects in a weight reduction program, the orientation of which was consistent with their generalized expectancies, would be more successful than subjects in a program inconsistent with locus of control beliefs. The volunteer subjects were randomly assigned to one of two weight reduction treatments, a self-directed program or a group program. The subjects were given two tests to determine locus of control: Rotter's I-E Scale and the Health Locus of Control Scale. The subjects whose locus of control orientation was consistent with the type of weight control program selected for them (self-directed program for internals or a group approach for externals) were significantly more satisfied with the program and tended to lose more weight than individuals whose locus of control orientation and treatment program were not consistent. Wallston, et al., (1976) found that classifying subjects as internals or externals on the basis of the Health Locus of Control led to results that were more congruent with the hypothesis than if the researchers had relied solely on I-E scores. This study provides valuable information for the classification of obese subjects to facilitate successful weight loss.

Wallston and Wallston (1981) studied 147 college students. They used five weight control programs in testing the hypothesis that, when given a choice, persons with an internal health-locus-of-control orientation would select weight management programs which were congruent with internal beliefs and that persons with an external orientation would choose externally oriented programs. The two externally controlled programs chosen by the fewest participants included hospitalization with a controlled diet and eating all of one's meals in a cafeteria where a fixed menu would offer no choices. No significant correlation was found between locus of control and choice of weight control program. Critique of this study includes noting that the subjects were not overweight.

Saltzer (1979) studied 115 women who began a clinic-based medical weight reduction program. Saltzer correlated Multidimensional Health Locus of Control scores and completion or noncompletion of a six-week program. Subjects also were administered a Weight Specific Locus of Control test developed by the researcher. Although there was not a significant difference in I-E scores between the completers and noncompleters, the scores of the completers were more internal on Saltzer's Weight Specific Locus of Control. Weight Specific Locus of Control internal subjects with high values on physical appearance or health were significantly more likely than other respondents to translate their behavioral intentions to lose weight into successful actions. The finding was specific to Weight Specific Locus of Control, not to the Multidimensional Health Locus of Control.

[*Since the researcher included the tools used in the studies she reviewed, the reader not only has a clearer picture of the relevance and usefulness of the findings, but also has the names of potentially useful research tools with references that should make it possible to obtain and evaluate the tool.*]

Tobias and MacDonald (1977) used a correlational study to determine the effectiveness of behavioral treatment in weight loss. They studied 100 undergraduate obese women and assigned them to one of five experimental conditions: weight reduction manual, self-determination alone, behavioral contract, effort control, and no control. The participants were tested for LOC orientation, using Rotter's I-E scale. Client responsibility without behavioral interventions was not found to be sufficient motivation for weight loss. Both behavioral intervention groups produced significant changes toward internality. The researchers concluded that this study further documents the effectiveness of behavioral programs. Both behavioral treatments in this study were executed in the absence of a therapist-client personal interaction.

Muhlenkamp and Nelson (1981) used a correlational design to study 36 newly enrolled clients in a commercial weight treatment program. They tested the hypothesis that subjects would become more internal as a result of weight loss. Each volunteer completed the Multidimensional Health Locus of Control Scale and a value scale that includes values of health and physical appearance. The subjects were asked to complete the same scales at the end of three months. Externally controlled subjects weighed more frequently at the weight center. Change towards internality was not positively correlated with weight loss. The researcher reported limited chances for any further shift in internality because of a highly internal sample.

Wineman (1980) used a retrospective design to study 116 members of Overeaters Anonymous (OA). He was interested in the relationship among locus of control, weight loss, and age at onset of obesity. The volunteer sample was obtained for convenience at an OA marathon. Volunteer participants were tested, using Rotter's Social Reaction Inventory Scale to measure locus of control and the Body Cathexis Scale (BC) to measure body image.

Adolescent-onset group members who were classified as old members had a larger weight loss and were more satisfied with their body images. A positive linear relationship between greater perception of internal control and a good body image was found in the entire adult-onset group. Results of the two-way analysis for locus of control according to onset of obesity and time enrolled indicated no significant effect on locus of control. There was minimal variation in the I-E scores among all the groups in this investigation. Although no significant correlation occurred between weight loss and locus of control, the researcher reported that the philosophy and program of the OA group might have biased the answers on both I-E and BC scales. The program supported the spiritual aspect of weight loss. Members were taught to rely on a "higher power" for help and guidance in weight loss.

Cohen and Alpert (1978) found externally focused obese patients to be at the highest risk for treatment failures. They studied 15 obese females who were employees of a New York University medical center. The volunteers agreed to be individually hypnotized weekly. A positive correlation was found between weight loss and internal control, as measured by Rotter's I-E scale. No significant correlation between level of weight loss and intensity of hypnotic trance was found.

Balch and Ross (1975) studied locus of control, using both a unidimensional and a multidimensional approach to study the completion and success in a self-control weight reduction program. They studied 34 volunteer females whose initial weights ranged from 127 pounds to 277 pounds. The treatment program consisted of nine weekly one-hour meetings, adhering to a behavioral format. Rotter's I-E scale (1966) was administered to all subjects at the initial group meeting. Of the subjects, 19 attended at least 75 percent of the meetings and were defined as "completers"; 15 failed to meet the criterion and were defined as "noncompleters." Subjects showing a weight loss greater than the median were considered "successes"; those losing fewer than 8 pounds were considered "nonsuccesses." Results indicated a significant correlation between internal Rotter I-E scores and both completion and success in the program.

[*The number of examples given here is extensive to illustrate two points: (1) the "field" should be reasonably extensively covered to give a fair overview of what is available and current in the area; and (2) the content covered in the various reviews is similar, but the writing style is easy to follow without being boringly repetitive.*]

Richard Stuart (1971) studied six overweight (171 pounds to 212 pounds), married, middle-class women, between the ages of 27 and 41. Each woman requested treatment on a self-referred basis. Treatment was offered on an individual basis; the women were assigned to one of two counselors. Both groups completed the Sixteen Personality Factor Questionnaire (Cattell and Eber 1967) and kept a record of weight and food intake for five weeks.

The first group was offered treatment twice weekly for 15 weeks. The second group was asked to practice "self-control." The same diet and exercise program was offered to both groups. The self-control group was not given instruction for management of food in the environment. Results of the study showed that patients in group 1 lost significantly more weight than those in group 2. Comparison of results of pre- and posttests of personality revealed little change other than small improvement in "ego stability." The results provide suggestive evidence for the usefulness of a threefold treatment of obesity, stressing nutritional planning, increased exercise, and environmental control of eating.

Leon and Chamberlain (1973) compared three groups of overweight persons (predominantly women): one group of 20 who had successfully maintained a weight loss over a one-year period; one group of 26 who had failed to maintain a weight loss; and a normal weight control group of 19 subjects. The overweight subjects were selected from a membership list of a local weight reduction club. All subjects had successfully dieted and had reached goal weight one year previously. The three groups were designated as follows: regainer group (26 females) had regained more than 20 percent of the weight previously lost; maintainer group (17 females, three males) had regained less than 20 percent of the weight previously lost; and the control group (18 females, one male) was composed of individuals who were either attending evening school classes or employed as office workers.

A questionnaire devised for this study provided detailed information about every circumstance in which eating occurred during a 24-hour period. The subjects were instructed to complete a questionnaire form on three different days. The subjects were told to designate a relative to observe and fill out a questionnaire recording the subject's behavior on one of the days. The subjects and the observers were instructed to work independently and to mail the completed forms to the evaluator.

The results supported the hypothesis that the type and amount of food eaten during mealtimes showed no significant differences among the three groups. The differences centered on between-meal eating, with the regainers showing a greater tendency to eat high-calorie foods in a greater variety of between-meal situations than the maintainer or control groups. Less activity outside the home was reported by the regainers. The regainers exhibited an association between eating and a number of daily activities and/or environmental cues unrelated to mealtimes, such as eating before bedtime, between meals, or while watching television. These results support previously reported findings that the obese are more responsive to external than to internal cues.

[*The last study reviewed does not use the term "locus of control"; however, the study is closely related to the locus of control literature by virtue of the common idea of individuals being greatly influenced by external cues (as in having an external locus of control). Useful studies do not have to deal directly with the current topic (or more accurately, the studies do not have to use identical terms) in order to be appropriately included in the literature review. There is a tendency for beginning researchers not to read broadly enough because they do not realize the usefulness of peripheral literature.*]

STUDIES OF CHANGES IN LOCUS OF CONTROL

Studies that do not directly deal with locus of control and weight loss provide information supporting the use of behavioral programs for weight loss. Parks, et al., (1975) studied 18 college students (ten females and eight males) who were desirous of eliminating self-defeating behaviors. An experimental design was used. Volunteer participants for a workshop were matched with a comparable control group. The workshop was based on the premise that individuals learn inappropriate coping behaviors in the process of maturing that become self-defeating. The purpose of the workshop was to prepare the participants to work through the fear of having to cope without dysfunctional coping methods. The participants were given Rotter's I-E once, with a follow-up test four months later. Participants became significantly more internally controlled than did the control group, as measured by the I-E scale. The main criticism of this study was the control group had not volunteered for the Eliminating Self-Defeating Behavior Workshop. This study does, however, support the hypothesis that locus of control can be changed.

A study by Dua (1970) illustrates information in support of a behavioral approach which may be helpful for weight loss. Dua used an experimental design to study three personality variables: extraversion, emotionality, and externality. His sample included 30 first-year female university students who expressed concern about their inability to relate in interpersonal situations. All participants in the study were receiving counseling at the university counseling center for this problem. In the experimental group, two subgroups were formed: a behaviorally oriented action program and a psychotherapy reeducation program. The control group received no treatment. The subjects received Rotter's C Scale and the Bendig Scale of Social Extroversion-Introversion and Emotionality. During the eight-week period, subjects of both the behaviorally oriented and the psychotherapy group met with a therapist for 30-minute individual sessions. The subjects in the experimental group reported that they had acquired more internal controls. Experimental subjects treated by the action program procedure had more changes along the dimension of internal-external control. The combined data from this study supported the specific hypothesis that action program procedures evoke significantly greater change than reeducation on the three variables studied.

[*Having completed the review, the researcher summarized the studies under an identifying subheading as illustrated below. The helpfulness of subheadings cannot be overemphasized, for they organize not only the reader but the writer. The summary informs the readers of what you have told them.*

The old admonition to "tell the readers what you are going to tell them" (introduction), "tell them" (content organized with identifying subheadings), and "tell them what you have told them" (summary) is still very sage advice.]

SUMMARY OF STUDIES

A number of researchers (Bulch and Ross 1975; Cohen and Alpert 1978; Saltzer 1979; Wallston, et al., 1976) have shown a positive correlation among internal locus of control, completion of a weight loss program, and weight loss. In other studies (Muhlenkamp and Nelson 1981; Wineman 1980), no significant correlations between weight loss and locus of control were found. In another study, subjects did not choose a weight loss program consistent with the individual's locus of control orientation (Wallston and Wallston 1981). Yet, another study showed that subjects who were assigned to weight control programs selected to be consistent with locus of control orientation were significantly more satisfied and tended to lose more weight than did subjects not matched to a weight loss group consistent with their locus of control (Wallston, et al., 1976).

Overweight individuals were found to be significantly more external in orientation (O'Bryan 1972). Behavioral treatment groups for the obese client (Stuart 1971; Tobias and MacDonald 1977) provided significant changes toward internality.

Studies not concerning weight loss (Parks, et al., 1975) further supported a shift toward internality and a behavioral approach for eliminating self-defeating behaviors. A behavioral approach (Dua 1970) for improving interpersonal relations was positively correlated with change toward internality.

Those who successfully maintained their weight loss (Leon and Chamberlain 1973) ate less between meals and had more activity outside the home.

This study was conducted to incorporate the positive changes of weight loss in the relationship to contextual shift by evaluating the internal-external control of participants in a weight loss group.

[Note that the researcher concluded the review of the literature by tying what had been done and reviewed to what she did.]

SUMMARY

After the review of the literature, you should be able to refine your question. Sometimes the question itself is not formulated in any way until after the literature has been reviewed. This approach would be true when there is something you have observed that "bothers" you and you are not quite sure how to put it into words. You go to the library or your general textbook on the subject for a start and get further interested and refine the problem from there. Whether you refine your research question or initiate it at this point, you should now have, in one sentence, a clear expression of what you want to study. In addition, you know who else has studied it, what they found, and what questions remain unanswered or are ready for some validation.

Following some suggestion for exercises and additional reading for literature reviewing, Chapter 3 provides explanations of theories, conceptual frameworks, and models.

Suggestions for Further Study

For the individual with an inquiring mind, the review of the literature can be exciting and filled with new discoveries. The problem will be to keep on the subject or change subjects systematically as indicated. Unfortunately, we often feel so pressured for time or get so caught up in completing assignments that we fail to recognize that what we are doing is actually enjoyable. Try the following exercises, preferably as a class or group assignment, so that you can share experiences.

1. Choose a question of interest. It may be the one you worked on in Chapter 1, or it may be a new focus. You are freer to explore, this time, because you do not have the constraint of having to find the phenomena to observe. The library is generally much more inclusive than our observational opportunities.
   a) Have any number of people find one reference on the question, make appropriate notes, and bring to class.
   b) Share the references by reporting what you found and having your peers question you about your source and information.

2. Summarize the information reported either as a written out-of-class assignment or have someone tie it all together at the end of class or report back to the group at the next class time.

3. Review the question. Does it still seem to be the focus of what you were really interested in or would you like to reword it? How is your question similar to what is in the literature reviewed? How is it different? If you did study the question you have posed, what would your findings contribute to the literature?

Suggestions for Additional Reading

Abdellah, F. G., and Levine, E. *Better Patient Care through Nursing Research* (2nd edition). New York: Macmillan Publishing Company, Inc., 1979, pp. 111–122.

Binger, J. L., and Jensen, L. M. *Lippincott's Guide to Nursing Literature: A Handbook for Students, Writers, and Researchers.* Philadelphia: J. B. Lippincott Company, 1980.

Brink, P. J., and Wood, M. J. *Basic Steps in Planning Nursing Research, From Question to Proposal* (2nd edition). Monterey, CA: Wadsworth Health Sciences Division, 1983. (Chapter IV)

Fox, D. J. *Fundamentals of Research in Nursing* (4th edition). Norwalk, CN: Appleton-Century-Crofts, 1982. (Chapter 6)

Gunter, L. "Literature Review," in S. D. Krampitz and N. Pavlovich (Eds.), *Readings for Nursing Research.* St. Louis: The C. V. Mosby Company, 1981.

McCloskey, J. C., and Swanson, E. "Publishing Opportunities for Nurses: A Comparison of 100 Journals," *Image,* 1982, *14*(2), pp. 50–56.

Polit, D. F., and Hungler, B. P. *Nursing Research: Principles and Methods* (2nd edition). Philadelphia: J. B. Lippincott Company, 1983. (Chapter 5)

Seaman, C. C., and Verhonick, P. J. *Research Methods for Undergraduate Students in Nursing* (2nd edition). New York: Appleton-Century-Crofts, 1982. (Chapter 6)

Chapter 3
How do others organize knowledge?

CONCEPTUAL FRAMEWORKS

Chapter Objectives

Upon successful completion of this chapter, the student will be able to

- Understand the value of conceptual frameworks for nursing research
- Identify the conceptual frameworks in reported research
- Suggest a conceptual framework or model for a topic of inquiry

INTRODUCTION

At the risk of seeming to divert from presenting the research process to a didactic discussion of abstractions, it is necessary to present some information that is new to many, if not all, undergraduate students. That is, the definitions of concepts, conceptual frameworks, and theories must be presented to form a base for discussion. Although the material is abstract and, therefore, difficult for some to appreciate fully, it is important for organizing thoughts and observations. You should not be troubled if you find other definitions or other approaches, for even your faculty may not agree among themselves or with the relationships of the terms presented here.

The term *conceptual framework* is used here in the same way that Fawcett (1984) defines conceptual model. The term *framework* gives a feeling of structure to support what one is trying to conceptualize. A conceptual framework is "a set of concepts and the statements that integrate them into a meaningful configuration" (Fawcett 1984, p. 2). Concepts are "words describing mental images of phenomena" (Fawcett 1984, p. 2). "A theory may be a description of a particular phenomenon, an explanation of the relationships among phenomena, or a prediction of the effects of one phenomenon on another" (Fawcett 1984, p. 19).

REASONS FOR APPLYING A CONCEPTUAL FRAMEWORK

Now it is possible that someone might question the necessity of going through all this effort to choose and apply a conceptual framework. In fact, researchers from other disciplines have belittled the tenacity with which nurses have adhered to the inclusion of a conceptual framework. Conceptual frameworks provide the source from which theories are derived. A theory is a higher order of conceptualization than a conceptual framework. Hypotheses are formulated from theories and are available for testing. Once a theory has been sufficiently tested to be proven, it is considered a law. Laws are rare, if they occur at all, in social sciences. Most laws are in the physical sciences—the Law of Gravity, for example. See Figure 3-1 for a summary of this organization.

Research is not conducted to merely answer one or a few questions. It is more than the testing of a hypothesis. Research is important for the development of a body of knowledge that can be called nursing and preferably uniquely nursing. For a more fully developed argument for the necessity of nursing research refer to Chapter 12.

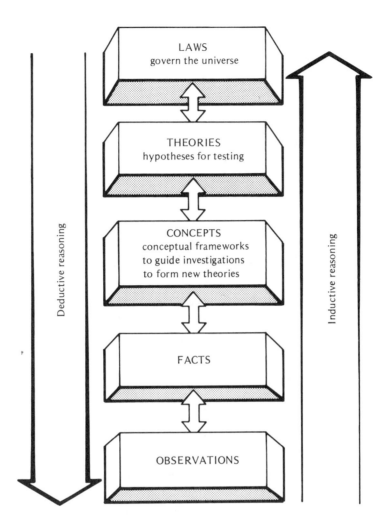

Deductive reasoning

Inductive reasoning

Figure 3-1. Building Blocks of Scientific Thought

Note in Figure 3-1 that you can think inductively or deductively. If you follow the steps in the order that the research process has been presented, from observations to formation of theory, you are reasoning inductively. An example of an inductive study is one reported by Lim-Levy (1982). "This study encourages review of the common empirical practice of changing temperature sites from the preferred oral to the less acceptable rectal or axillary sites in patients receiving oxygen inhalation treatments" (p. 150). The study is based on observation and practice; it is not generated by theory. The results may contribute to the questioning of current theory or to the generation of some new concepts, but the stimulus for the study is experience and observation.

You can organize your thoughts in the opposite way. You can start with a theory and deduce what you would expect to observe. Hallal (1982) based her study of "The Relationship of Health Beliefs, Health Locus of Control, and Self-Concept to the Practice of Breast Self-Examination in Adult Women" on a theoretical framework consisting of three elements: the Health Belief Model, the construct of health locus of control, and self-concept theory. Based on this framework, Hallal generated the following hypotheses:

1. The health belief scores of adult women who practice breast self-examination will be higher (i.e., will reflect greater perceived susceptibility and greater perceived benefits) than the health belief scores of adult women who do not practice breast self-examination.

2. The health locus of control scores of adult women who practice breast self-examination will reflect a higher degree of internality than the health locus of control scores of adult women who do not practice breast self-examination.

3. The self-concept scores of adult women who practice breast self-examination will be higher (i.e., will reflect higher self-concept levels) than the self-concept scores of adult women who do not practice breast self-examination (p. 139).

Hallal designed the study to test these hypotheses, which were generated from the theoretical framework. Thus, Hallal's study is an example of deductive reasoning.

Arguments have been developed to imply that one way of thinking was "better" than the other. It is best to avoid value judgments (recognizing that this statement is a value judgment), and maintain an objective attitude in all aspects of research. Maintain a questioning attitude, one that says, "Show me." The philosophers of the Middle Ages were using deductive reasoning when they debated the number of angels that dance on the head of a pin. Skinner (1950), on the other hand, advocated inductive reasoning when he asked, "Are Theories of Learning Necessary?"

Following the research process as outlined in this text, the identification of a problem area precedes the choice of a conceptual framework. Experienced researchers, however, tend to "live" with a conceptual framework which dictates, for them, the direction of the research process. You may, therefore, choose a conceptual framework from which you develop a research question, or you may find a conceptual framework that supports your research question.

CONCEPTUAL FRAMEWORKS FOR RESEARCH IN NURSING

At the same time as you are reviewing the research that has been done on the question you identified, you begin to think about the question in a broader context. What are the concepts related to your question? A concept is an idea, a word, a conceptualization or an experience, a thought, or an observation. If you are interested in nutrition in neonates, the concepts might be physiology of the newborn, feeding patterns, metabolism of the newborn, mother-infant relationships and impact on nutrition, symbiosis of mother and infant, chemical elements in mother's milk versus cow's or goat's milk, dependency, or any number of others. Start by considering all possible concepts you can think of or find that relate to your research question. Which of those concepts seem to fit better than others? Do some reading and thinking about the ones you choose. Now how do they fit? Narrow the field to a few (three to six, if you insist on numbers), and identify some constellation that they seem to form. Usually, the concepts will remind you of some conceptual framework or theory you have previously encountered—from nursing or from some other field.

Many conceptual frameworks from other disciplines have been applied in nursing studies, and currently there are a number of nursing models from which to choose. Theories from authorities outside of nursing include systems theory, adaptation theory, stress theory, social learning theory, behavior theory, and the health belief model. Nursing models include Johnson's Systems Model, Roy's Adaptation Model, Orem's Self-Help Model, and Rogers' Life Process Model. The following discussion provides an overview of selected conceptual frameworks with applications to nursing studies.

Systems Theory Applied to a Nursing Study

Systems theory has been expounded by von Bertalanffy (1968) to involve elements composing subsystems which combine to form systems that, in turn, can be combined to form suprasystems. A system can be open or closed. A closed system does not permit anything to enter or leave the system. In contrast, an open system is one that takes in nutrients, information, or other substances from the environment, and returns something to the environment (waste or information, for example). The environment is whatever surrounds the system. Systems theory is as simple or as complex as you want to consider it. On its simplest terms, consider input as food, the system as a living organism, and output as waste. Note that all living organisms are open systems. On a more complex basis, a human being is composed of many systems: digestive, neuromusculoskeletal, integument, genital, endocrine. Several human beings combine to form a system known as the family. Families form communities that form societies. So which is the "system"? The system of interest is the component you define as the system in your study.

Sablay (1981) was interested in individuals who had problems with alcohol. After working in an inpatient detoxification unit and an outpatient clinic, Sablay noted that many of the clients who were detoxified and referred to the outpatient unit never kept their appointments and later (but not much later) were readmitted to the inpatient unit to repeat the detoxification process. Sablay defined the client as the system and thought that if the appropriate feedback were received, the client could be redirected to give a different output, specifically, to keep appointments in the outpatient clinic, abstain from the further use of alcohol, and cease the need for readmission to the detoxification treatment unit. The benefits are obvious: an individual is reclaimed from a cycle of self-destruction and need for expensive health care to being potentially a healthy person.

Stress Theory Applied to a Nursing Study

Stress theory was developed by Selye (1976). Stress theory includes the concepts that individuals respond to stressors in the environment in general ways. Depending on the inherent vulnerability of the individual, some specific part of the body may begin to show more deterioration than others in the face of continued stress. One of the most interesting concepts to emerge from stress theory is that pleasant events such as holidays, weddings, and promotions, are stressful and have the capacity to produce physiological reactions.

Talmadge (1982) used stress theory to provide a framework for her study of impaired nurses. Talmadge thought that nursing is a stressful job. The nurses, who had joined a rehabilitative program for impaired nurses with an addiction to either alcohol or some other drug, were considered to have sought relief from the stresses of nursing by using drugs. Within this framework, Talmadge designed her study to try to identify whether indeed stress had been a contributing factor to the initial use of the addictive substance.

Social Learning Theory Applied to a Nursing Study

Social learning theory has been used in a number of nursing studies. There are several approaches within the broader context of social learning theory: locus of control, modeling, and role theory. Locus of control refers to the source of decision making for an individual. Some individuals seem to be controlled from within—they make decisions independent of what is going on around them; others, who are considered to be outwardly controlled, are prone to be fatalistic. Those controlled from within have an internal locus of control, and those who believe they have little control over what happens to them have an external locus of control.

The weight control study, from which the literature in Excerpt 2-1 in Chapter 2 was taken, used locus of control as the conceptual framework. Locus of control has also provided the framework for studies of women and the practice of self-breast examinations (Hallal 1982).

Modeling, another concept from social learning theory, is an effective approach for teaching individuals new behaviors. Children can be taught to imitate or model the behaviors of other children, a nurse, a teacher, a researcher, or most anyone. In her study of the effects of sex education, deLemos (1975) used the modeling of the instructor as a framework. The instructor exhibited knowledge of sexual behaviors, and she did so with ease and poise. The framework of modeling predicted that the participants of the workshop would be able to model the desirable behaviors of the instructor. It turned out that there was a significant difference in the sexual knowledge and attitudes of the participants following the workshop as compared to their knowledge and attitudes prior to the experience.

A Nursing Model Applied to Nursing Research

Martha Rogers (1970) has developed ("is developing" is more accurate) a comprehensive model of nursing which has the potential for broad applications. Rogers' model was applied in a study of the sexuality of elderly confined to an intermediate care facility.

EXCERPT 3-1 _____

SEXUAL ATTITUDES, KNOWLEDGE, AND BEHAVIORS
IN A GROUP OF NURSING HOME RESIDENTS

CONCEPTUAL FRAMEWORK

Martha Rogers' model of the unified wholeness of man (1970) constituted the conceptual framework underpinning this study. Rogers identified several fundamental attributes of man which contribute to the formation of a set of "basic assumptions on which nursing science builds" (p. 47). The basic assumptions presented by Rogers include:

1. "Man is a unified whole possessing his own integrity and manifesting characteristics that are more than and different from the sum of his parts" (p. 47).
2. "Man and environment are continuously exchanging matter and energy with one another" (p. 54).
3. "The life process evolves irreversibly and unidirectionally along the space-time continuum" (p. 59).
4. "Pattern and organization identify man and reflect his innovative wholeness" (p. 65).
5. "Man is characterized by the capacity for abstraction and imagery, language and thought, sensation and emotion" (p. 73).

Man and the environment are viewed as energy fields characterized by openness, wholeness, pattern, and organization. Energy fields have no boundaries, and therefore, extend to infinity (Rogers 1980).

Rogers stated, "human and environmental fields are continuously characterized by wave pattern and organization but the nature of the pattern and organization is always novel, always emerging, always diverse" (1980, p. 331). She further theorized that the energy fields of man and the environment are patterned as a spiral and may be diagrammatically represented using the model of a "Slinky" (Figure 1).

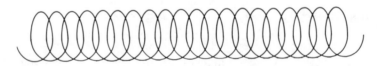

Figure 1. Diagrammatic Representation of the Energy Fields of Man and the Environment, Using the Model of a "Slinky"

The energy field of each man is similar in its spiralling pattern, yet different in the variations of that pattern. For example, the spirals of the model may run close together, far apart, and at various angles from each other (Figure 2). The same is true for environmental fields.

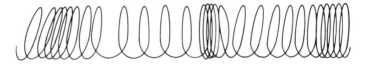

Figure 2. Diagrammatic Representation of the Variations in the Pattern of an Energy Field

The uniqueness and diversity of the sexual needs of each aged individual can be depicted using this model.

Rogers' (1970) homeodynamic principle of synchrony, which is derived from the previous assumptions, has special applicability to the study of patterns of sexual attitudes, behaviors, and knowledge of nursing home residents. According to Rogers, the principle of synchrony is: "Change in the human field depends only upon the state of the human field and the simultaneous state of the environmental field at any given point in space-time" (p. 98). The concepts of pattern and organization are inherent in this principle. Therefore, the pattern of sexual attitudes, knowledge, and behaviors of nursing home residents would reflect the mutual, simultaneous interactions occurring on the biological, psychological, and sociocultural levels between the environment and the residents. Rogers stated, "pattern and organization take on greater complexity as life evolves" (p. 99). In addition, she wrote, "the particular pattern that identifies the human field at any given point in space-time is unique" (p. 98). This would imply that the sexual patterns of thought, behavior, and knowledge of institutionalized elderly individuals would be unique to them alone, reflect a greater complexity than existed in earlier years, and be indicative of their special needs and concerns. Rogers herself acknowledged the applicability of the principle of synchrony to the aging process when she stated, "This principle is in contradiction to an all-too-common practice of interpreting various behavioral manifestations in adults as equivalent to developmental behaviors occurring in an earlier developmental stage" (1970, p. 98). In a more recent publication, she expressed that "aging is a continuously creative process directed toward growing diversity of field pattern and organization. It is NOT a running down" (Rogers 1980, p. 336). It is, therefore, inappropriate to speak of "regression" or to refer to an elderly individual as being "like a child."

The author of the above excerpt emphasized the actualizing of the elderly individuals in their spiralling progression toward equifinality. As you reread the excerpt, notice that the application of a conceptual framework to a research problem requires an integration of the concepts that make up the framework with the variables to be studied. It is not acceptable simply to identify the theory and leave it to the reader to make the connections.

A list of research topics and accompanying conceptual frameworks that might be used for the investigation of each topic appears in Table 3-1.

TABLE 3-1
Research Topics with Possible Conceptual Frameworks

TOPIC	CONCEPTUAL FRAMEWORK
1. Compliance in taking hypertensive medications	1. Health belief model *or* Behavior modification
2. Support for grieving relatives of ICU clients	2. Grief and grieving *or* Crisis intervention
3. Stress management for ICU nurses	3. Selye's stress theory *or* Coping strategies
4. Management of hypertension of pregnant clients	4. Physiology of hypertension *or* Biofeedback
5. Exercise effects on elderly clients	5. Physiology of exercise *or* Self-esteem
6. Maintenance of body temperature in premature neonates	6. Systems theory *or* Heat radiation physics

Notice that each topic has two possible conceptual frameworks listed. There are other possibilities. Some frameworks are borrowed from social or physical sciences. Although the trend is for nurses to develop nursing conceptual frameworks, it is still important to recognize the usefulness of concepts from other fields and apply such concepts appropriately. Besides, some of those theories from other fields may be the ones you are more comfortable with at this time; familiar theories, such as developmental theory, physiological concepts, and learning theories, are easily applicable to nursing research problems.

SUMMARY

Conceptual frameworks for nursing research are important as they provide organization and direction for research. Although nurses have borrowed concepts and theories from other disciplines, a growing number of nursing models are proving to be useful. After some suggestions for further learning and additional reading are presented, Chapter 4 will deal with basic research terms called "variables."

Suggestions for Further Study

The more you work with the abstract concepts of nursing models and related theories, the more comfortable you will become with the ideas. The following exercises are designed to help you develop familiarity with conceptual frameworks.

1. Discuss which conceptual framework would fit the problem you have identified. If you cannot match your problem with one of the frameworks described in this chapter, what concepts are you concerned with? What would you need in order to have a useful framework? Can anyone find one?

2. When you have identified what seems to be an appropriate framework, describe how it relates to your problem. If possible, what would be predicted on the basis of the framework you have chosen? You can relate framework to problem by taking the concepts of the framework and describing how those concepts (taken one at a time) translate into the problem.

3. Once again discuss whether you wish to modify your question based now on the conceptual framework. Resolve any discrepancies between the question, the literature, and the conceptual framework.

4. From the following list of articles with clearly identified conceptual frameworks, choose one or two that interest you, review it (them), and report back to your study group.

ROLE THEORY

Young, K. J. "Professional Commitment of Women in Nursing," *Western Journal of Nursing Research,* 1984, *6*(1), pp. 11–26.

SYSTEMS THEORY

Beck, C. T. "Parturients Temporal Experiences during the Phases of Labor," *Western Journal of Nursing Research,* 1983, *5*(4), pp. 283–295.

THE BETTY NEUMAN HEALTH CARE SYSTEMS MODEL

Ziemer, M. M. "Effects of Information on Postsurgical Coping," *Nursing Research,* 1983, *32*(5), pp. 282–287.

PHYSIOLOGICAL MODEL

Farr, L., Keene, A., Samson, D., and Michael, A. "Alterations in Circadian Excretion of Urinary Variables and Physiological Indicators of Stress following Surgery," *Nursing Research,* 1984, *33*(3), pp. 140–146.

Suggestions for Additional Reading

Fawcett, J. *Analysis and Evaluation of Conceptual Models of Nursing.* Philadelphia: F. A. Davis, 1984. (especially Chapter 1)

The Nursing Theories Conference Group. *Nursing Theories: The Base for Professional Practice,* Englewood Cliffs, N.J: Prentice-Hall, Inc., 1980. (Chapter 1)

Polit, D. F., and Hungler, B. P. *Nursing Research: Principles and Methods* (2nd edition). Philadelphia: J. B. Lippincott Company, 1983. (Chapter 6)

Riehl, J. P., and Roy, C. *Conceptual Models for Nursing Practice* (2nd edition). New York: Appleton-Century-Crofts, 1980. (Chapters 1 and 2)

Chapter 4
What are you going to look for?

IDENTIFICATION OF THE VARIABLES

Chapter Objectives

Upon successful completion of this chapter, the student will be able to
- Identify variables in research questions
- Classify variables in terms of their relationships to the research questions
- Define variables operationally as they relate to specific studies
- Describe the formulation of hypotheses as indicated by the research questions and classification of the variables
- Identify tools for measuring variables
- Discuss the validity and reliability of measurements of variables
- Differentiate between controlled and uncontrolled variables

INTRODUCTION

By now you have identified something that you want to investigate. You have gone to the library and reviewed the resources related to your interest. You have thought about the concepts involved, reviewed relevant resources, and related your project to the theory or model that will serve as your conceptual framework. Of course, you have applied your project to nursing. You are now ready to narrow your focus to variables. Table 4-1 summarizes the types of variables that need to be identified.

IDENTIFYING THE VARIABLES
IN THE RESEARCH QUESTION

Identifying your research variables is as important as stating your research question. In fact, each very clearly relates to the other. The variables are the observable, measurable phenomena that you propose to study. As the term implies, the phenomena must vary in some way: presence or absence, amount or type. Having identified the research variables, you must indicate what role they play in your study. Research variables may be broadly classified as independent and dependent variables.

TABLE 4-1
Variables

---

1. *Research variables*—identifiable from research question and/or hypothesis. Research variables include

   a) *Independent variables*—also called experimental, treatment, causal, or stimulus variables

   b) *Dependent variables*—also called criterion, effect, or response variables

   c) *Correlated variables*—neither dependent nor independent, but occurring in the presence of each other

2. *Extraneous variables*—all relevant variables that are not the direct focus of inquiry; that is, they are not identified in the research question or hypothesis. Extraneous variables include

   a) *Environmental variables*—factors which impinge on the individual (economic, anthropological, sociological, and physical factors)

   b) *Organismic variables*—physiological, psychological, and demographic factors

---

Independent Variables

The independent variable is the variable that is observed, introduced, or manipulated in order to determine what effect it has on another variable of interest (the dependent variable). Depending on the research approach (discussed in Chapter 5), the independent variable may be called more appropriately the experimental, treatment, causal, or stimulus variable.

In a descriptive study, you may be observing a phenomenon to determine whether it occurs with some regularity before the occurrence of some other phenomenon. For example, you may observe two-year-old children to determine whether they cry less frequently during immunization injections when the parent holds the child than when the child is held by the nurse. Assume that you do nothing to change what is already occurring in the clinic, you are not manipulating or treating or changing anything—you are merely observing events that are occurring in the environment. The independent variable is who holds the child—parent or nurse. The dependent variable is crying—absence or presence. Because we are looking at the event in this sequence, there is the *implication* that who holds the child "causes" crying. You could reverse the order (sequence): If the child is crying, is the mother more likely to hold the child? In this question, crying is the *independent* variable—the variation being absence or presence of crying behavior. Who holds the child becomes the *dependent* variable, the implication being that the child's crying "causes" the one person more frequently than the other to hold the child.

An experimental research approach, in which the researcher randomly assigned a random sample of two-year-old children to be held by the parent or the nurse while receiving an injection, might lend more credibility to the concept of cause as associated with the independent variable. While cause is sometimes used synonymously with independent variable, you should maintain skepticism of "causation" when doing research with people in complex environments.

The terms *experimental* and *treatment variables* refer to the independent variable in experimental studies. The terms experimental and treatment are synonymous in this context. You should not confuse experimental treatment with clinical treatment of clients, although in many instances they will be the same. Treatment, in the research sense, means manipulation, not necessarily therapeutic procedures (although certainly never evenly potentially harmful). A research "treatment" might be the use of audiovisual feedback in the simulated practice of interviewing techniques.

The term *stimulus variable* makes sense in the context of stimulus and response events. Likewise, the term *antecedent variable* is also used inter-

46

changeably with that of independent variable. While the use of so many different terms is confusing and there are sometimes shades of differences among the terms, further complicated by lack of consistency among researchers to use them in any standard way, the independent variable *must* precede the dependent variable.

Dependent Variables

The dependent variables are probably the most interesting variables in the study. These are the phenomena you observe for change or reaction after you apply the treatment or observe the occurrence of the independent variable. As is true with independent, there are several terms that are used as synonyms for the term *dependent variable:* criterion, effect, or response variables. *Criterion variables* are those variables in studies in which the purpose is to determine the effect of the independent variable by predetermining the criterion that must be reached in order for a decision to be that a change has occurred. For example, in a study to motivate elderly individuals to participate in an exercise program, the criterion as to whether subjects exercised might be that they attended eight of the ten available sessions.

Use of the term *effect* for the dependent variable makes sense if you use the term *cause* for the independent variable. Likewise, if the independent variable is referred to as the *stimulus variable,* the dependent variable is appropriately termed the *response variable.* The term applied to the dependent variable should correspond to the term used for the independent variable. The dependent variable *must* occur after the independent variable.

Correlated Variables

There are studies in which the researcher is not interested in which variables occur first or which occur after the other variables. The researcher is interested in how dependably the research variables occur together. The relation of chronic mental illness and lower socioeconomic level is an example of correlated variables. There is a high correlation of poverty and mental illness; that is, the incidence of mentally ill individuals is greater among the population within the poverty income level. This fact does not imply that poverty "causes" mental illness or that mental illness "causes" poverty—there is simply a high correlation. To name one of these variables as the independent and the other as dependent is illogical (although some researchers do it). The research question in this case would be stated in terms of *relationships:* for example, what is the relationship of mental illness and poverty?

DEFINITIONS OF TERMS

In order to keep research precise, the research variables must be unambiguous. Scientifically speaking, terms have meaning only within particular theoretical contexts. The meaning of the terms should clearly reflect your conceptual framework. If you choose to combine one or more conceptual frameworks for your study, you must be even more careful to make your definitions precise so that they do not fall ambiguously between the frameworks. Terms that need to be defined include the variables and the key theoretical terms or concepts.

The variables must be precisely defined according to the meaning they have in the study. If the levels or classes of your variables are easily identified (such as males and females), you have an easier task than if they are given to a wider possibility of interpretation (such as short, long, heavy, or fast). Even so, these latter variables can be measured by generally acceptable measuring instruments such as rulers, scales, and speedometers. All you have to do is specify that "long" is between three and three-and-one-half inches, "heavy" is anything over 200 pounds, and "fast" is running a mile in six minutes. Those measures are fairly clear to everyone. Your definitions need to be consistent with common usage and be professionally useful in order to be meaningful to colleagues and others with whom you wish to communicate. Everyone does not have to agree with you, for you define the variables to fit your study; however, your study will get more attention and be more meaningful if you use language and criteria that are consistent with the literature and practice. Your definitions must be consistent with your conceptual framework or you have chosen the wrong conceptual framework.

Suppose you are interested in self-esteem, body image, attitudes toward elderly individuals, or sexual identity. How are you going to measure these variables? First, you must define what *you* mean by the term. In order to do so, you may choose from any number of sources: a dictionary, an authority either in nursing or some other discipline. The conceptual framework for your study is one of the best sources of an operational definition. Tools for measuring variables are frequently developed from the conceptual framework. You may narrow, combine, or broaden your definition. The point is that you must make clear what you are studying. For example, body image may be defined as the composite of attitudes one has about one's body parts. You may then define "composite of attitudes," "body parts," or even separate "composite" and "attitudes." Obviously, that is a bit cumbersome, and it is not clear that you or your readers would know what you were studying after you had completed that exercise. Another option is to indicate that you are defining body image as stated, and that it will be measured by, say, the Secord-Jourard Body Cathexis Scale. You must make sure that you are measuring what you say you are measuring by selecting a tool that is valid for the variable you wish to study.

Some researchers differentiate between operational and theoretical definitions. It may be preferable to combine them, as in the example of the body image measurement. You may define body image as "how one perceives one's own body parts" (conceptual definition) "as measured by the Secord-Jourard Body Cathexis Scale" (operational definition).

FORMULATION OF HYPOTHESES AND/OR IDENTIFICATION OF STUDY QUESTIONS

Now, you are ready to either formulate an hypothesis or to identify some study questions. Hypotheses go with cause and effect studies or experiments or where the literature review supports a specific prediction. Study questions go with descriptive and correlational studies and where relatively little evidence to support a prediction exists.

Hypotheses

If you wish to study causes and effects of variables, it will be appropriate for your study to have an hypothesis. If you are describing stimuli and responses, you probably want to have hypotheses. If, however, you are describing antecedent and following events or studying the correlation of variables, you may not wish to formulate hypotheses.

A *research hypothesis* is a statement of expectation of outcome of the study and generally states a direction of the expectation. For example, clients who receive preoperative teaching will have *less* pain than clients who receive no preoperative instruction. The null hypothesis is a statement that is tested by a statistical analysis. As the term *null* implies, the null hypothesis is a statement that there is "no difference" when the independent variable is present or manipulated. Stated in this way, the statistics are applied in order to disprove (or reject) the null hypothesis. (Statistical testing of hypotheses will be discussed in Chapter 7.)

The hypothesis includes the research variables as they have been identified and defined. The researcher states formally how these variables are presumed to relate. The statement is written in future tense and is usually preceded by a stem such as "This study will be conducted to test the following hypothesis: Surgical patients who receive preoperative teaching will ex-

perience less postoperative pain than similar patients who receive none."
The researcher may have a primary hypothesis with several subhypotheses
which will provide data for testing the primary hypothesis. An example of
subhypotheses might be:

> This study will be conducted in order to test the hypothesis that pa-
> tients who receive preoperative teaching will have a healthier post-
> operative recuperative period than patients who do not have such
> instruction. In order to test this hypothesis the following subhypoth-
> eses will be tested. When compared to a similar group of subjects,
> postoperative patients who receive preoperative teaching will

1. Require less pain medication
2. Spend fewer postoperative days in the hospital
3. Tolerate a regular diet sooner
4. Exhibit fewer symptoms of emotional distress

Hypotheses are particularly useful when you have a hunch you want
to study. That preconceived idea becomes your hypothesis and your research is designed to test it.

Study Questions

If you are more vague about the relationship of the variables of interest to
you, you may be at a descriptive stage and the research question may be
more appropriate until more is known about those variables. As with the
hypothesis, the major question may be stated in general terms with specific
subquestions to guide your research. Your question might be, "What is the
relationship between locus of control and weight loss among a group of
women in a weight loss program?" Subquestions to guide the study might
be

1. Will subjects who are more internally controlled lose more weight
   than those who are externally controlled?
2. Will the direction of the locus of control change with successful weight
   loss?

Measurement of Variables

The measurement of variables refers to how you collect the data about the
variables in order to test the hypothesis or answer the research question.
Some variables are easy to measure. For example, you can easily *count* how
many students come to an extra class designed to prepare for final exami-

nations. If, however, you wish to determine if the class made a difference in grades for those who came, you have a different kind of measuring to do; you would probably compare the grades of those who attended the extra class with those who did not.

Even when you are using seemingly objective measuring tools such as thermometers, scales, and rulers, you must recognize that all are not standardized accurately. Use the same scales, if possible, for determining the weight of subjects. Use the same type of thermometer and temperature site for measuring temperatures. Thermometer and blood pressure readings vary among those doing the readings. Keep the number of individuals collecting the data to a minimum and check to see how nearly they agree on the measurements on the same subjects at the same time (reliability checks between or among data collectors). Have all data collectors follow precisely the same procedures and calibrate the equipment frequently.

Measuring attitudes (toward elderly individuals or clients with various health problems) or emotions (happiness, depression, anxiety) becomes a challenge. There are tools developed for measuring these variables. The trick is to identify and obtain the appropriate tool to measure the variable. The tool must be designed to measure what you want to measure in order to be *valid* for your study. The tool must also be *reliable;* that is, using it must consistently provide the same information on the same subject under the same conditions. In other words, assuming that the anxiety of the subject has not changed, a reliable tool would yield the same level of anxiety for the individual on Friday as it did the previous Monday. If using the tool does not produce a very similar score when conditions have not changed, the tool is not reliable.

Research tools include questionnaires, scales, inventories, surveys, and checklists. These tools may most readily be found in studies similar to yours and in the conceptual framework. The description of the tool in the source should include tests for reliability and how validity has been established. Note that a test that is appropriate for one population might not be appropriate for another. Choose a tool that has been done on a population as similar to yours as possible. (More about reliability and validity is presented in Chapter 6.)

The question frequently arises about constructing a new tool, such as a questionnaire, for one's own study. There are three good reasons why this practice is not encouraged: (1) it takes a great deal of time to develop a questionnaire; (2) it requires fairly sophisticated statistical procedures to establish validity and reliability; (3) since the purpose of research is to contribute to a body of scientific knowledge, the contribution is potentially greater if the data are collected with tools used by others so that results can be more easily compared. Try, whenever possible, to use standardized tools. When none are available, be prepared to work closely with an experienced researcher and statistician in developing a new instrument. Data collection sheets where you list events and record observations are more easily developed, but must still be carefully thought out and systematically constructed. Pretesting is advised for even the simplest of data sheets because surprises do occur and the more you uncover before you are committed to the study, the fewer frustrations you will have during the study.

EXTRANEOUS VARIABLES

Extraneous variables are all relevant variables that are not the direct focus of inquiry. These variables include all that are not identified in the research question or hypothesis. While these variables are not the primary focus of your study, they cannot be ignored for they may influence the outcome of your study. The theoretical framework and related research studies provide you with information about potential extraneous variables. Extraneous variables include organismic and environmental variables (Abdellah and Levine 1979).

Environmental Variables

All of the factors which impinge upon the subjects are classified as environmental variables. Examples of environmental variables include: climate, family composition, governmental organization, work organization, physical setting, ideological climate, and community setting (Abdellah and Levine 1979). If you are studying the reactions of clients to being seen by a nurse practitioner in a health maintenance organization, a rural setting might yield different data than an urban setting. Subjects from colder climates might have different health problems when compared to subjects in warmer regions.

Organismic Variables

Included in variables classified as organismic are age, sex, marital status, education, type of work, personality, height, weight, blood pressure, racial group, nationality, religion, job skill, intelligence, hair color, eye color, political belief, income, and level of wellness (Abdellah and Levine 1979). Attitudes on a variety of subjects, health problems, and other dependent variables will tend to differ with variations in the organismic variables.

Control of Extraneous Variables

Extraneous variables may be either *controlled* or *uncontrolled*. When variables are controlled, the researcher has taken some measures in the design (planning) of the study to prevent the variables from having a biasing influence on the outcome of the study. Controlling variables may be done in any of several ways.

1. Random sampling (to be discussed in Chapter 5), to ensure that there is no bias in the selection of the subjects from the group being sampled, is useful.

2. Limiting the sample to subjects having specified organismic characteristics (such as ages 40 years through 50 years or all males) narrows the focus of the study. The advantages are that the data will be specific to populations having that (or those) characteristics. The disadvantage is that the results may be generalized (applied) only to the population for which the sample was representative.

3. Having subjects serve as their own controls is desirable in many studies, especially experimental ones to determine a before and after treatment effect.

Uncontrolled Variables

Sometimes the researcher recognizes that, in order to obtain a reasonable sample, it is necessary to compromise. (In fact doing research is like building a house: you have a wonderful idea but, due to limited time, funds, and availability of materials, you modify the design until what you come out with is not what you originally had planned to build.) If, for example, you wanted to compare the housing preferences of elderly individuals living in one geographic location with the preferences of a similar group living elsewhere, it would be desirable to study individuals who were either as nearly alike as possible or were proportionally representative of the groups you wished to study. It would be delightful if the subjects could be matched on age, sex, living arrangements (identical neighborhoods), identical histories (including whether married, number of years married, same number of children, same work conditions, etc.), identical incomes, and other social indices. Depending on how strictly you defined these variables, you would have a limited number of available subjects. The number of variables on which subjects are matched must be small, or the researcher will have a small sample due to inability to find pairs that match. Therefore, the researcher announces that some variables which could conceiveably or theoretically influence the data are uncontrolled in this study.

Uncontrolled variables should be kept to the minimum that is possible while still obtaining an adequate population within the constraints of the researcher's resources. When control of extraneous variables in sampling is not possible, the effects of these variables can be analyzed statistically in order to determine the influence exerted by the variables in question. The point is that as long as you are interested in studying human beings, there are likely to be difficulties in getting homogeneous samples. You simply must recognize the limitations of your study and design the best project possible.

Mediating Variables

You will not find agreement on the definition or importance of mediating variables. It is not necessary that you concern yourself very much with this concept at this time; it is included here for your convenience in finding a discussion if you have heard of it or read of it elsewhere. As the name implies, mediating variables are those that go between other variables and in some way facilitate the connection. For example, if one has an insufficient fluid intake (by some reasonable measure), one is thirsty. Think about it—a number of physiological processes occur within the body between the event of fluid need (lack of fluid replacement) and a subjective feeling one identifies as thirst. Compare a study of the relationship of SAT scores and successful completion of college. Millions of events occur in the life of a college student, any of which might have some influence on the completion of college. If a student has a terminal illness and never makes it through college, what does that have to do with the SAT score made before entering college?

So what do you do about mediating variables? There are several possibilities, from ignoring them to controlling for them. If age of first pregnancy seems to make a difference, you can include age in your research variables, have everyone in the study approximately the same age, or list the lack of conformity on age as a limitation of your study. You run into a lot of trouble as far as being able to draw any inferences from your data if your experimental sample is one age and your control sample is another. Research designs are developed in order to deal with these various problems related to the handling of variables. This problem will be dealt with in more detail in the next chapter.

SUMMARY

Variables are what you are studying plus what might confound (confuse) or otherwise influence what you are studying. The relationship of the variables must be specified in order for the study to be understood. The research variables must be defined in such a way as to be measurable. The definitions must be clear enough that interested researchers may repeat the study accurately.

Suggestions for Further Study

1. Obtain a recent copy of a nursing research journal and find the hypothesis of a study reported. Identify the variables. What is the independent variable? What is the dependent variable? Are any controlling or confounding variables apparent? Check your answers by reading the article. The variables should be appropriately identified in the text of the article.

2. Identify the independent and dependent variables in the following hypotheses:

   a) Following abdominal surgery, clients who receive primary nursing care will recover at a faster rate than clients who receive team nursing care.

   b) Hyperactive children who have no added sugar or artificial coloring in their diets will learn more efficiently than hyperactive children who have unrestricted diets.

   c) Middle-aged women who are on Diet A will lose weight faster than middle-aged women who are on Diet B.

3. Which terms in the hypotheses listed in #2 need to be operationally defined? Operationally define at least two terms in each hypothesis.

4. Identify and define the variables in the problem you were working on in Chapter 1 and/or Chapter 2.

Suggestions for Additional Reading

Abdellah, F. G., and Levine, E. *Better Patient Care Through Nursing Research* (2nd edition). New York: The Macmillan Company, 1979. (Chapter 7)

Brink, P. J., and Wood, M. J. *Basic Steps in Planning Nursing Research, from Question to Proposal* (2nd edition). Monterey, CA: Wadsworth Health Sciences Division, 1983. (Chapter VII)

Chapter 5
How do you plan to do it?

RESEARCH DESIGNS

Chapter Objectives

Upon successful completion of this chapter, the student will be able to

- Differentiate between two major research approaches
- Give examples of research designs consistent with each approach
- Give rationale for random sampling
- Use a table of random numbers to randomly assign subjects to two or more experimental groups
- Discuss the relationship of each type of design to theory building
- Choose appropriate designs for studying a variety of research questions

INTRODUCTION

If designing a study seems formidable, take courage. Your first design might take considerable thought, revisions, and criticisms (constructive, hopefully). A dozen designs later, you will not even remember how difficult the first one was. An experienced researcher will have a repertoire of designs from which to choose. Learning to design a study is simply a matter of carefully and logically planning and putting into words or a flow chart on paper what you plan to do. A design is a blueprint or detailed plan.

Research designs may be divided into two broad approaches: experimental and nonexperimental. (Some researchers categorize designs differently, but not necessarily inconsistently with the organization suggested here.) The term *approach* is used to indicate, in a general sense, how you are going to attack the problem. That is, are you going to do something and see what happens (experimental) or investigate what is or has been (nonexperimental). The term *descriptive* may be substituted for nonexperimental and is more frequently used. If you manipulate one or more variables, your approach is experimental; if you do not do anything to any variables, your approach is descriptive. It is imperative that your approach is appropriate for your research question. Given that the question is relevant and timely or has value by some criterion, if the approach fits the question, it is a good research approach.

Under each approach is a variety of designs. A design is a detailed plan of how you are going to implement your approach. Several designs are used so frequently that they are named, and the reader will have a good idea of how the research was done just by the name of the design (e.g., quasiexperimental, survey, or comparative).

Each approach contributes to the development of a body of nursing theory. Lindeman and Schantz (1982) have identified building blocks of research theory (Figure 5-1). Surveys and descriptive and exploratory designs form foundations and rationale for designing experimental studies. Experimental studies must be replicated (repeated on the same or other populations) in order to develop confidence in the findings. The consistent findings of replicated research then lead to theory.

Although experiments enjoy greater prestige in some circles, the novice investigator should not assume there is something inherently better about experiments.

If no descriptive studies exist, it is premature to conduct an experimental study. Unfortunately, some researchers are so intrigued with experimental studies that they use them prematurely. Untimely

choice of experimental design can produce results that have no statistical significance without the support or an understanding of the
actual cause and effect relationship. (Lindeman and Schantz 1982, p.
10)

In a field such as nursing, with little research produced as part of planned
research programs, many areas still need careful description.

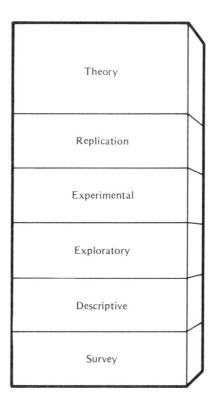

Figure 5-1. Building Blocks of Research Theory

SOURCE: Lindeman, C. A., and Schantz, D. "The Research Question." *The
Journal of Nursing Administration,* January 1982, pp. 6–10.

EXPERIMENTAL APPROACH

As indicated, an experimental approach is one in which some variable is
manipulated in some way. A "true experimental design" meets the three

criteria of manipulation, control, and randomization (Polit and Hungler 1983). A "quasiexperimental design" lacks either randomization or control (or both). A "preexperimental design" includes some manipulation of one or more variables but no control group, randomization, or adequate numbers of subjects for generalizations. A case study is an example of a preexperimental design. More information on the three types of experimental designs is presented in Tables 5-1, 5-2, and 5-3.

Suggestions for Strengthening Experimental Designs

In a preexperimental study, one could add something to the environment and see if it made a difference. For example, if you place a fresh flower on the breakfast tray of a depressed patient, what will the response be? Obviously, many terms must be defined in this question, but it is an experimental question because the researcher is doing something to the situation that is not being done prior to the study. Let's suppose that we clarify what we mean by a fresh flower and where and how it will be placed on the tray. (If it is wilted by the time it gets to the patient, it may have the opposite of the intended effect.) Let us also suppose that we appropriately define what we mean by "depressed" patient. We have to have some indication of what the responses of the patient are before the "treatment" (what the experimenter does to the subject). What those responses are is known as the *baseline*. The same measure must be used and measured at the same time of day and under the same circumstances in order to compare the *posttreatment* responses with the *pretreatment* responses, and determine if, indeed, there has been a change. (Whether any measurable change is significant is another consideration and will be discussed in detail in Chapter 7).

Suppose we use the Beck Depression Scale given to the patients at 6 P.M. the evening before the "treatment." We then place a fresh flower on the tray of the patients each morning for five mornings, repeat the administration of the Beck Depression Scale, and compare the latter with the first findings. We find that the scores are consistently in the direction of less depression. What, if any, conclusions can be drawn? If you say "none," you are correct. Why?

Adding Control Groups

All we know is that the patients in our study are consistently less depressed (at least on this scale) than they were five days previously. We don't know why. We have to consider whether administering this scale to the same subjects within such a short time period is appropriate for that scale. That

TABLE 5-1
True Experimental Design

Definition. A true experimental design is characterized by (1) manipulation; (2) control; and (3) randomization.

Purpose. The purpose is to determine if manipulation of the independent variable(s) has an effect on the dependent variable(s).

Advantages. True experimental designs produce the most convincing evidence concerning the cause and effect relationship between variables. Hypotheses are required in experimental studies.

Limitations. The limitations of true experimental designs include

1. Some variables are not manipulable
2. Ethical restrictions (as withholding drugs or treatments)
3. Practical restrictions (as prohibitive costs)

TABLE 5-2
Quasiexperimental Design

Definition. A quasiexperimental design is an experiment that lacks either (1) randomization or (2) control group or (3) both.

Purpose. The purpose of a quasiexperimental design is the same as that of a true experimental design, i.e., to determine if the manipulation of the independent variable(s) has an effect on the dependent variable(s).

Advantages. The advantages of the quasiexperimental design, especially as compared to the true experimental design, are

1. Practicality
2. Feasibility
3. Generalization ("to a certain extent")

Disadvantages. The disadvantages of quasiexperimental studies is the possibility of other interpretations of the findings, such as

1. History (differences due to time)
2. Selection (e.g., volunteers are a biased sample)
3. Maturation (e.g., developmental changes)
4. Testing (subjects may learn from the test tool)
5. Mortality (subjects dropping out of the study)

TABLE 5-3
Preexperimental Design
Example—Case Study*

Definition. A case study is an indepth investigation of an individual, group, institution, or other social unit. Implied in the classification as an experimental approach is the assumption that the researcher is manipulating some variable in the "case."

Purpose. The purpose of a case study is to analyze and understand the variables that are important to the history, development, or care of the subject.

Advantages. The advantages of a case study are

1. The generation of information which may lead to the formulation of hypotheses for further study
2. Clarification of concepts and variables for further study
3. Elucidation of ways to measure the variables

Disadvantage. The primary disadvantage of preexperimental studies is the inability to generalize the findings to a larger population.

---

* A case study might be a descriptive (nonexperimental) study if the researcher merely observes or collects data in some other way without influencing the variables.

is, is it still reliable? Is there a practice effect? (A practice effect is doing better on subsequent trials as a result of previous experience on the same task.) Even if the scale is still accurate, we have questions. How do we know that the patients did not improve just because of the nature of the illness? Depressions usually lift after a period of time. What about medications the patients are taking? Sometimes medications are effective. Then, there is always psychotherapy and milieu therapy that might have some influence on the patients' behavior. Note that these other factors, which might be responsible for the change in the dependent variable, are the alternate explanations referred to in Table 5-2 under disadvantages of quasiexperimental designs.

When questions of this nature are asked of students, the students have been observed to look rather hopeless and ask "How do you ever do anything?" Without being melodramatic, it is very important to develop a questioning attitude. Just because a would-be researcher does something and measures some change does not mean the change is necessarily the result of the treatment.

So, what do you do about your project? How can you determine if in fact your fresh flowers do have an effect? A control group will help. If you have two groups who are "matched" on all identified characteristics you could give all the members of one group flowers and not give the other group members flowers and determine if there is a difference. (You still have the problem of the practice effect of the tool, but for the present assume your measurement is appropriate.) If you find that the group who got the flowers had decreased in their depression more than the other group, are you sure it was the flowers that made the difference? No, it might have just been the extra stimulus of having something put on the tray.

Right! You are going to need another group. Have one group in which you place the fresh flower on the tray; a second group in which you place something else on the tray such as a menu, or name card, or some other stimulus that is an addition to the regular items on the tray. Then you have a control group, for which you do nothing. Now, test the subjects to determine if there is any difference.

There are further considerations. How long should you continue to place the flower before you retest? Is the original thought of five days long enough? How long are patients on this unit usually hospitalized? How much is it going to cost you to obtain the flowers? Are you going to include men and women, or do you think that women might respond more readily to flowers than will men so in the interest of expediency you choose to include only women? Comparing the responses of men and women (the sex difference question) could be another study.

Random Assignment

Suppose you have now decided to make the study last for two weeks. You observe, however, that it is next to impossible to match subjects on all of the important characteristics. What do you do? Make *random assignments* to groups. This assignment could be done by putting the names of all the available patients into a hat and drawing them out. The first one drawn would be put into group 1 (the group who gets the flower); the second name drawn would be put into group 2 (the group who gets the menu on the tray); and the third name drawn would be placed in group 3 (the group who gets no treatment). The fourth name drawn would be placed in group 1 and so forth until the desired number of subjects has been placed in each group or until the available sample has been exhausted.

Random assignment is a technique for minimizing the effects of uncontrolled variables. For example, if all the patients in B wing were in one group and all the patients in Y wing were in another group, the differences found between the two groups might be due to something that is different about the two wings rather than to your treatment. Another example is if you have all adolescents in one group and all adults in the other group, any differences might be due to a developmental stage rather than to an experimental (or treatment) effect.

Random Sampling

Random assignment and random sampling are two phases of the process of organizing your subjects into research groups. Random sampling is done when the population of potential subjects who meet your criteria for being in your study is greater than the number of individuals you can study. That is, they have the characteristics you have determined are important for your investigation. It may be that they have the right disease or are from the right socioeconomic class, are the right age, or the appropriate birth order—whatever you are studying. Assume, for example, that you are studying high school seniors. Your criteria include being currently enrolled in high schools that have student bodies of more than 400. You plan to include all of the high schools in your state that meet this stipulation. You want a fair representation, but your budget does not permit you to include all 3,000 students who are seniors in the local high schools with total enrollments of more than 400 each. You need to obtain a sample of this population. In order to get a fair representation, you will select your sample randomly. Two ways of random sampling are (1) have a computer print out all names that qualify, cut them into equal-sized pieces of paper, and draw them out of a container; and (2) let each number from one to 3,000 equal a name, go to a table of random numbers, and choose the first 400 numbers that occur. The names which correspond to the numbers will be your sample.

Table of Random Numbers

Using a table of random numbers (see Appendix D), choose a place to start—any place—it is your choice. Decide whether you will progress forwards or backwards (or sideways or from bottom to top—random tables are fun). Also decide whether you will choose every digit, or every other digit, or whatever you like. From your 3,000 high school students, you want to have 400 for your sample. Number each member of your population.

From your random number table choose the first four digits at a time from each entry (or the last four). For example:

59034
25630
14027
00463

Throw out the 5; there are not 5,903 individuals in your population, so you cannot use that one. For 2563 identify that individual as "No. 1" and place that one in group 1. Number 1402 from your population will be your second subject, and will go in group 2, and number 46 from your population will become your next subject in group 1. You continue until each of the 400 members of your sample has been randomly selected for your study sample. When you come to a number that you have already assigned, simply disregard it and go on to the next item in your list of random numbers.

Although a simple example has been used for clarity, given the case cited, it would be more expedient to number the members of the population in the order of the random table. Since the order of odd and even numbers would be random in a list of random tables, you would then have a random assignment if you put all of the odd-numbered members in group 1 and the even-numbered members in group 2 until you have 200 in each group.

Why can you not just go down the list of members of the population and put every other one in group 1 and the others in group 2? You probably could in most cases and come out with groups as similar as you would using the random numbers technique. However, there are possibly some spurious circumstances in which that would not work. For example, if you went into a classroom where the teacher has arranged the students so that boys and girls alternated, you would come out with all boys in one group and all girls in the other. The same problem might occur in a hospital. Suppose you chose the patients in every other room; every other room might be private, with alternate rooms being four-bed wards. You might not be willing to assume for your study that patients in wards respond the same on your research variable as do patients in private rooms. There are any number of reasons that there might be differences—patients in private rooms might be more acutely ill, they might be from a different socio-economic background, they might have different physicians, the nurses might prefer to care for patients in the ward because it is easier to care for them in that setting than going into private rooms. The point is that there are great possibilities of spurious samples if they are drawn systematically rather than randomly from the population. Again, a spurious sample is one that does not accurately reflect the population from which it is drawn.

Suppose that you want to study something about nurses. The population of your study is all registered nurses in the United States. However, your budget does not permit you to contact each of the approximately 2 million members of the population. How can you sample the population so that you stay within your budget and still have a representative sample? (This is a real life problem.) If you take all nurses from a given state, there might be something unique about that particular state. If you choose all nurses who are members of the American Nurses' Association, you have another self-selected group, for the ANA has a membership of about one-tenth of the total population of nurses. You might guess that the membership of ANA is different in some way from the nurses who have not chosen to be members of their professional organization (a worthy topic for study). With a project of this magnitude, you are likely to have access to a computer that could randomly select the sample for you according to the characteristics you determine. The point is that you want to randomly sample, meaning that every member of the population has an equal chance of becoming part of your sample. The reason for random sampling is to keep down the possibility of any findings being due to some peculiarity of the sample rather than being something that can be generalized to the population as a whole.

Stratified Sampling

To complicate things somewhat, let's go back to the high school population. Suppose you were not content to leave the selection entirely up to chance because it is important to you that you have an equal number of girls and boys and an equal number of students from each grade (high school freshmen, sophomores, juniors, and seniors). Obviously, you will divide 4 (the number of grades) into 400 (the number desired for your sample). Then, for an equal number of boys and girls in each grade, you will want 50 boys and 50 girls from each grade level. The process for obtaining the 50 from each subpopulation of freshmen boys, freshmen girls, sophomore boys, and so forth is the same as if you were getting the number from the entire population. That is, you will number each member of the subpopulation and draw from your table of random numbers the first 50 whose numbers appear. You now have an example of *stratified sampling*, or a sample which has a predetermined distribution of subsamples.

Stratified sampling is frequently used in research with human beings because there are frequently subpopulations with characteristics that need to be considered in analyzing any findings. In the previous example of all registered nurses, any number of subsamples might be desirable depending on the nature of your study. If you are interested in regional differences, you might want an equal number from each designated geographic region. Or, you might want an equal number of nurses from each of the three traditional, basic educational programs—diploma, associate degree, and baccalaureate degree. Note that in this latter example you are eliminating some registered nurses, including those from generic master's programs in nursing and those from external degree programs. Whether or not you want to do so depends on your study—the purpose and the kind of generalizations you want to be able to make about your findings.

With any design, from the simplest to the most complex, the help of a consultant is valuable. Sampling is a complicated concept, and appropriate sampling techniques demand advanced statistical expertise. Never hesitate to consult an expert whenever one is available. Most requests for research money include consultation fees in the budget.

Nonrandom Sampling

All studies are not based on random sampling of subjects. Some studies are done on *volunteers* and pose some questions as to what you can say about the findings. (Note that a design that does not include randomization is not a "true" experimental design. If it includes manipulation of any of the variables, it is either "quasiexperimental" or "preexperimental.") Are nurses who volunteer for a study the same in important characteristics as those who do not volunteer? By no means can you put all those who volunteer into one group and those who do not volunteer into another group and make some comparisons or state that the nonvolunteer group is a control group.

Other studies are done on a *convenience* sample, or one that is available at the time the researcher wants to collect data. There are problems in using convenience samples which make it difficult to generalize the findings. For example, if the researcher uses the critical care nurses who work days in the university hospital where the researcher is a faculty person, can the researcher generalize the findings about those particular nurses (symptoms of burnout, for example) to other critical care nurses who work other shifts or rotating shifts in that hospital, to critical care nurses in other university hospitals, to the hospital nurses in the region, or to other nurses in the community? There are no universally accepted rules about what generalizations might be made. There are, however, some conventions that apply. In general, you cannot generalize beyond the population of the sample you have studied. Without random sampling, you cannot generalize beyond your *sample*. This rule should not discourage you or other nurses. You should be aware of the limitations of any study you design, read, participate in, or critique; but no design is perfect. You do the best you can with your resources at the time of the study and recognize your limitations. In addition, you must remember to be realistic about your conclusions.

Incidentally, to *generalize* means to make statements about the entire population based on the findings from your study. The generalizations you might make also depend on the statistical analysis of your study. Statistics will be discussed in more detail in Chapter 7.

You will read in reputable journals research articles that report on studies that were done using samples selected systematically or conveniently. There might be a shade of difference between the two terms: Systematic sampling would be predetermining that your sample will consist of every second or fourth patient who comes into the clinic who otherwise meets your research criteria; convenience sampling would be taking the first predetermined number of clients who present themselves for services at the research site. Another example of a convenience sample is one which includes clients who are admitted to an inpatient psychiatric clinic during a specified time period. Even though you may design or participate in such studies, you should be aware that those sampling techniques are a compromise. Sometimes the choice is to sample conveniently or not do the study. If the study is important, and if it will provide some new information or confirm some findings from previous studies, it is important; the compromise is acceptable.

Why do we talk about compromise in sampling when we discuss nursing studies? Why not just do tight, precise designs and quit hedging? It is without apology that we are interested in people. People are found in a great many places that are hard to control experimentally. That is not a value judgment; that is a fact. We need to accept that fact and plunge full speed ahead and design the very best studies possible to get the most information available under the circumstances.

The Nature of Experimental Designs

Experimental designs range in complexity from very simple to exceedingly complex. As defined earlier, experimental designs are those designs in which the independent variable is manipulated. These designs are helpful in looking for answers to questions of: Does the initiation of variable x into a situation change variable y in the situation? Does the removal of x have an effect on y, or does increasing or decreasing x have an effect on y? Obviously, x has to be defined, and y not only has to be defined but the effect to be observed (measured) has to be indicated.

The simplest design is the pretest-posttest in which you gather information about a variable, do something to the subject (called *treatment*—in the research sense, not referring to health care), and gather information about the variable after the treatment. For example, you can give a test to a class (pretest) to see how much they know about a subject; give them the information by teaching a class or making an assignment (treatment); test them again (posttest) to determine if, in fact, they have changed in their ability to perform on that particular test.

Why not just provide the treatment (teach the class) and give a test? You would know how much the subjects knew according to their performance on that test, but you would not know how much they had learned from the treatment. They may have already had the information; in which case the treatment was not necessary. This is an example of a quasiexperimental design because it lacks both randomization and control; however, if this design had not had a pretest, it would be an example of a preexperimental design. The addition of a control group and random selection and assignment would make the design true experimental.

The rationale for including a control group to improve the design is that without the control group, you cannot be assured that any difference between the pretest and posttest is because of the treatment. There are several reasons individuals may change—*maturation, catastrophic events,* or something else going on in the lives of the subjects. Maturation means that the individual is different because of being older and the process that accompanies growing up or growing old. For example, if you measured and weighed five-year-old children (thus obtaining a baseline, which is the same idea as a pretest) and then put them on a special diet for two years to determine the effects of this diet, what would differences in weights and heights mean? Essentially nothing, because you expect children to grow taller and gain weight between their fifth and seventh years.

In order to overcome the maturation and other problems encountered with the pretest-posttest design, you can use a control group and compare the differences between the control group and the experimental or treatment group. With this design, you could determine if the gains in heights and weights of the group you fed the special diet were greater than those of the group to whom you did nothing. Suppose you do get a difference, can you be sure that the difference was due to the diet? Not necessarily. There is the well known "Hawthorne Effect," which seemed to indicate that the changes in one population were in fact due to the attention they received rather than to the treatment (manipulation of schedule) which was the independent variable. So the difference in the children who got the diet might have been due to the attention of having a special diet rather than to the diet itself.

Use three groups: one gets the special diet; the second gets a "placebo" (that is, gets something that looks like the special diet and receives the same amount of attention, but does not contain anything that would be a dietary supplement—or in any way harmful); the third group would get nothing. You would expect that groups two and three would be similar in results, with group one showing greater gains than either of the other two groups. A refinement of the design would be to have two experimental groups—one that gets more of the special diet than the other to determine if there is a correlation between the amount or strength of the special diet and growth. You may find that those subjects on the greater amount became obese—too much of a good thing.

NONEXPERIMENTAL (DESCRIPTIVE) APPROACH

When using a nonexperimental or descriptive approach to research, the researcher does not manipulate any of the variables. Instead, the researcher is interested in describing what is (descriptive design) or what was (documentary-historical design). Survey is another term used for descriptive designs that are focused on the present. If the description compares two or more groups, the design is *descriptive comparative*. If the description is concerned with the relationships of two or more variables, the design is *descriptive correlation*. There are variations and nuances of each of these designs; some designs combine two or more types. These classifications are guidelines for thinking through your procedure and for considering the approach taken by others in research you read or in which you participate. Tables 5-4, 5-5, and 5-6 summarize characteristics of three types of nonexperimental designs.

Strengthening Nonexperimental Designs

Sampling, choice of measurements or observation tools, and precision in data collection are just as crucial in nonexperimental designs as they are in experimental designs. The sampling techniques described under experimental designs also apply to nonexperimental studies. It may be even more important in nonexperimental designs to have a larger sample and to have a "representative sample," one that has approximately the same proportion and distribution of important variables as the population you wish to describe.

Nonexperimental studies are not easy. They require careful review of the literature, much thought and integration into a conceptual framework, and careful collection of data. If done correctly, and in order to be meaningful, large amounts of data may be generated requiring sophisticated statistical analysis. These admonitions are not meant to discourage you, but only to encourage you to plan carefully in order to design a meaningful study.

TABLE 5-4
Documentary-Historical Design

Definition. A documentary-historical design involves systematic collection and critical evaluation of data relating to past occurrences.
Purposes. The purpose is to test hypotheses or answer questions concerning causes, effects, or trends relating to past events which may shed light on present behaviors or practices.
Advantages. Documentary-historical studies allow the researchers to investigate an event which is unlikely to be duplicated.
Disadvantage. Subjectivity is the chief disadvantage. There is danger of biases in selection of data.

TABLE 5-5
Survey

Definition. A survey focuses on the status quo of some situation, and data collection is directly from the sample.
Purposes. Surveys are designed

1. To describe (percentages and averages may be used)
2. To explain (variables of interest are explained by examining relationships)
3. To predict (to forecast future outcomes)
4. To explore (to begin inquiry where little is currently known)

Advantages. Positive characteristics of survey include flexibility and broadness of scope.
Disadvantages. Inferences regarding causal relationships may not be made.

TABLE 5-6
Descriptive Correlation Design

Definition. A descriptive correlation study is designed to determine how variables change in terms of one another; an increase in the magnitude of one is associated with a change (either increase or decrease) in the other (Seaman and Verhonick 1982).

Purpose. The purpose of a descriptive correlational design is to describe relationships among variables.

Advantages. Advantages include

1. An effective and efficient means of collecting a large amount of data about a problem area
2. Data are collected in the natural environment and are therefore more generalizable than studies done in artificially controlled settings.

Disadvantages. The disadvantages of the descriptive correlational design studies are

1. Variables are not manipulated, so control is not in the hands of the researcher.
2. Causal relationships may not be inferred.
3. Because of the lack of control of variables, interpretations may not be accurate.

Discussion of Nonexperimental Designs

A researcher proposes to describe the influence of a neighborhood "root worker" on the health care of the community. The historical individual died about 60 years ago, but the researcher believes that there are survivors who remember the root worker and can describe the influence she had on the lives of the survivors, their families, and the community. Some of the practices and teaching of the root worker may be influencing health care today in that community. The sources of data are interviews with the survivors, diaries of contemporaries, newspaper clippings, and other public documents. Obviously, this proposal is an example of an historical research design. The researcher will not have a hypothesis, for there is no prediction; research questions will be posed to guide the study. Such questions might include the following. What newspaper clippings of the era included references to the root worker? Of individuals who knew her, what do they recall of their relationship to her? Whom did she treat? What methods did she use? Are any of these methods still being used in that community today? By whom?

Another example of a proposed historical design was one to study the relationship of the development of psychiatric-mental health nursing specialists and legislation related to mental health and nursing education. This study, too, would include interviews with individuals who were involved in the developments and historical documents. The purpose of the study was to determine if a relationship between legislation (particularly as relates to funding) and nursing education could be found.

A study designed to describe the characteristics of a group of nurses in treatment for problems with alcohol and/or drug abuse is an example of a survey to describe characteristics of the sample. The method of data collection included structured interviews with the members of the group. Study questions included the following. Did the nurse perceive herself or himself to be under stress at the time of beginning chemical use? What are some common health and personality characteristics? What precipitated the nurses seeking treatment? What suggestions do the nurses have for preventing and treating others who have similar problems?

An example of a descriptive correlational study is one that was designed to examine the relationship of locus of control and weight loss. The question was whether the amount of weight loss was correlated with degrees of locus of control. This study is an example of one that is sometimes confusing to classify, for something was, in fact, done to the subjects; that is, a treatment was applied. The subjects were in a weight reduction group. The researcher, however, was not responsible for the group. Therefore, the researcher merely *described* what was; she did not manipulate anything and, therefore, had no control over the treatment variable. The group was one of a series of offerings in a community noncredit educational program. The weighing was a part of the program.

We are all familiar with surveys through the mass media, in classrooms, in communities. Surveys may be as mundane as how many people use a certain toothpaste. Some surveys are important; for example, health care or child care needs in a community. Obviously, you can do a simple survey by asking your colleagues what they believe to be the most critical issues in nursing. You may learn something about your colleagues, but you certainly may not generalize that knowledge to other groups. Well-designed surveys are needed and challenging to conduct.

SUMMARY

Research designs are the blueprints developed by the researcher to guide the research. Two research approaches are experimental (the independent variable is manipulated) and nonexperimental or descriptive (no manipulation of variables is done). Within these two approaches are a variety of research designs. Choice of design depends on the careful consideration of the advantages and disadvantages of each in relation to the purpose of your study and the research question you have formulated.

Implementation of the research design involves the collection of data. The collection of research data is the focus of the next chapter.

Suggestions for Further Study

As previously indicated, you will learn more if you have the opportunity to discuss the questions below with peers. There may be more than one possible answer for some, and a discussion of the advantages and disadvantages of various responses is recommended.

1. Consider each of the research questions below and decide which research design, from the list given, you would choose. What are the advantages and disadvantages of the design you chose?

   Designs: True experimental
   Quasiexperimental
   Preexperimental
   Descriptive survey
   Descriptive correlation
   Historical-documentary

   a) What are the characteristics of prenatal women who choose to attend Lamaze childbirth classes?

   b) What was the relationship of governmental legislative and financial support and the development of graduate programs in psychiatric nursing?

   c) What are the effects of intensive case management on the hospital recidivism rates of chronically mentally ill individuals, as compared with a similar group who do not receive intensive case management?

   d) What are the attitudes of clients toward nurse practitioners providing care in a prepayment health maintenance clinic?

   e) In a sample of adult women, what is the relationship between locus of control and persistence in an exercise program?

f) What is the effect of family therapy on the adjustment of a family in which the father has been diagnosed and treated for neurosyphillis?

2. Identify the appropriate design for the research question you have formulated. Have your design critiqued by your peers and refine it as indicated. Where would you do your study? What is the population? How would you select your sample?

3. From a real or imagined population, select a random sample using three methods: a) drawing names (or numbers) from a hat (or bag); b) flipping a coin (or rolling dice); and c) using a table of random numbers (Appendices A–D). Compare the characteristics of the samples chosen by the three methods as to how representative each sample is of the population. For example, if 30 percent of the population is female, which sampling method gave you the closest to 30 percent females in the samples?

4. Considering the design you chose for your study, what would be the contribution of the findings to theory building? What would the next step be after completion of your study?

Suggestions for Additional Reading

Fox, D. J. *Fundamentals of Research in Nursing* (4th edition). Norwalk, CN: Appleton-Century-Crofts, 1982. (Chapters 9–12 and 18)

Isaac, S., and Michael, W. B. *Handbook in Research and Evaluation.* San Diego: Robert R. Knapp, Publisher, 1971.

Lindeman, C. A., and Schantz, D. "The research question," *The Journal of Nursing Administration,* January 1982, pp. 6–10.

Polit, D. F., and Hungler, B. P. *Nursing Research: Principles and Methods* (2nd edition). Philadelphia: J. B. Lippincott Company, 1983. (Chapters 8–11 and 19)

Seaman, C. C., and Verhonick, P. J. *Research Methods for Undergraduate Students in Nursing* (2nd edition). New York: Appleton-Century-Crofts, 1982. (Chapters 8 and 9)

Chapter 6
How do you stick to your plan in the real world?

RESEARCH PROCEDURE AND METHODS

Chapter Objectives

Upon successful completion of this chapter, the student will be able to

- Describe an appropriate research procedure for investigating a problem
- Describe several research methods
- Identify research methods appropriate for selected research designs
- Describe criteria for evaluating research tools
- List potential sources of error in data collection

INTRODUCTION

Collecting the data is probably the most exciting part of the research process. After so many hours (days) in the library reviewing literature and searching for the appropriate conceptual framework, it is a welcomed relief to get involved in the actual data gathering activity. There are two important phases of data collection: planning the collection and following the plan. As you have probably guessed, it is not quite as easy as it sounds.

PLANNING THE DATA GATHERING PROCEDURE

Planning involves thinking through in detail, step by step, exactly what you must do to collect the data (the units of information) to answer your research question or test your hypothesis. Start with getting permissions and include what method you will use for collecting the data. An example of proposed research is included in Excerpt 6-1.

EXCERPT 6-1 _____

LOCUS OF CONTROL AND SUCCESSFUL WEIGHT LOSS

PROCEDURE AND DATA GATHERING PROCESS

Before conducting this research, permission will be obtained from the faculty thesis advisory committee and the Human Investigations Committee for the School. Before approaching the weight reduction class, the researcher will obtain permission from the psychologist teaching the class. At the first class meeting, the researcher will explain the study and ask for volunteers. The participants will be assured that individual identities will not be revealed. Each volunteer will be requested to sign a Subject Consent Form (Exhibit 6-1). Demographic data will be requested on the Demographic Data Questionnaire (Exhibit 6-2), and locus of control will be assessed by the Adult Nowicki-Strickland Internal-External Locus of Control Scale [*a copy was included in the proposal*]. The demographic variables—age, sex, education, living situation, meal preparation, familial history of weight problems, other attempts at weight loss, and physical activity—were chosen to examine the similarities of the sample in this study to other overweight populations in other studies.

Exhibit 6-1

(Name of School)

SUBJECT CONSENT FORM

Title of Study: Locus of Control and Successful Weight Loss

My name is _____. I am a registered nurse conducting a study on weight loss as part of the requirements for a Master of Nursing degree. I am interested in the differences and similarities among individuals in weight control programs.

If you agree to participate in this study, your weight and height will be measured. You will be given a questionnaire asking your opinion on topics in a variety of areas and a questionnaire concerning your personal background.

Your signature on this consent form will give your permission to participate in the study. You will be reweighed at the end of the six weeks of class and asked to complete a similar questionnaire.

Your name will not be used at any time in the description of the study. You will not benefit directly from this study.

Your participation or nonparticipation in the study will not affect your involvement in this weight loss program.

I understand that I may make any inquiries concerning this study.

I understand that I am free to withdraw my consent and to discontinue participation in the study at any time.

I hereby consent to participate in this study.

Date	Signature of Subject

Witness	Signature of Investigator

This consent form includes no exculpatory language through which the subject is made to waive any of his/her legal rights and to release the institution from liability for negligence.

Signature of Investigator

Exhibit 6-2

DEMOGRAPHIC DATA QUESTIONNAIRE

1. Name_____

2. Age (circle one): under 20   21–30   31–40   41–50   over 50

3. Sex (circle one): Male   Female

4. Highest level of education (circle one):

   8th grade or less   9th-11th grade   High school graduate

   Some college:_____ years completed   College graduate

   Postgraduate study—highest degree held: _____

   Technical or specialty education (specify): _____

5. Are you presently living alone? (circle one):

   Yes   No

6. Who prepares majority of meals? (circle one):

   Self   Other

7. Who in your family has had or now has a weight problem? (circle one):

   Mother   Father   Both mother and father   Neither mother or father

8. How many times have you sought group assistance for weight loss? (circle one):

   Never   Once   Twice   More than twice

9. What is the largest amount of weight you have lost at one time? (circle one):
   0–5 lbs.   6–10 lbs.   11–15 lbs.   16–20 lbs.   More than 20 pounds

10. How often do you participate in physical activities (skiing, gardening, jogging, swimming, aerobics, etc.)? (circle one):

    Daily   3 times per week   Weekly   Seldom or never

The Adult Nowicki-Strickland Internal-External Locus of Control Scale was selected as a tool for measuring locus of control because of the criticisms found in the literature of the Rotter (1966) Internal-External LOC Scale. Criticisms of the Rotter scale included the following: difficult language for the noncollege-educated adult, scores affected by social position (Nowicki and Strickland 1982).

The Adult Nowicki-Strickland Internal-External (ANS-IE) was presented in 1972. The scale consists of 40 items that are answered either yes or no. Nowicki and Duke (1974) tested the discrimination validity of the scale by investigating the relationship of the ANS-IE scores to social desirability. Consistent with the requirements of discriminate validity, ANS-IE scores were not related to scores from the social desirability measure ($r = 0.10$). Test-retest reliability was reported by Nowicki and Duke after they studied college students ($n = 48$) over a 6-week period ($r = 0.83$).

The subjects will be weighed on a floor model scale. Subjects who complete the 6-week course will be retested by repeating the ANS-IE scale and weighing on the same floor model scale used at the beginning of the study. All tests will be administered and scored by the researcher and weights will be recorded by the researcher.

Repeatability of the Study

The criteria for evaluating the procedure is to ask: "With the information given, could I repeat this study just as the researcher did it?" In the example presented, perhaps you could come close, although there would be some questions about the population—criteria for being designated as "overweight," the nature and setting of the class, the role played by the psychologist leading the class, how the class had been advertised or whether members were referred by their physicians, or what incentives might have been used to promote weight loss.

Obtaining Permissions

The steps of the study are clear. Permissions will be obtained from the student's thesis advisers, the person conducting the weight reduction class the researcher proposes to use, the appropriate Human Investigations Committee, the authors of the research tool, and the subjects. Much more about ethics and research may be found in Chapter 11 of this text. At this point, we are talking about procedures rather than the philosophy and rationale of ethical considerations that are the bases for obtaining consent.

Permissions from Authorities and Authors

Although verbal consent from the psychologist conducting the class and the authors of the ANS-IE might suffice, written consent is always preferable and more assuring. A letter to the authors of a research tool is usually all that is required. Simply state in the letter what you are researching, how you plan to use the tool, and ask for permission to do so. Usually the author of the tool will not only grant permission to use the tool, but might include an updated version and a bibliography of articles in which the use of the tool was mentioned. Also, the author typically will request the data from your study to add to the data already collected. The pooled data will help to broaden the generalizability of the tool.

Subject Consent

Look at Exhibit 6-1 for an illustration of some of the elements of a consent form. The researcher identifies herself by name and position. It is important that the subject have that information to know who the researcher is (whether a nurse or a research assistant or a liberal arts major or whoever) and why the researcher is doing the study. Potential subjects usually trust nurses, so that appropriate identification is not only ethical but facilitative.

The consent form contains a list of exactly what is expected of subjects. The information could have been more explicit about the estimated amount of time a subject would need to complete the questionnaires. The time of the repeat of the measures is stated and confidentiality is promised. Note also that the subject is told that participation will not benefit the subject in any way. This statement is considered necessary so that subjects are not deceived into thinking that they will be paid for participation or that other rewards might be forthcoming. Assuring subjects that neither participation nor nonparticipation will affect their program, whether academic, health care, or other, is important, and the researcher must adhere to that promise. No coercion whatsoever is allowed.

The subject has the right to ask questions (and get truthful answers). The subject also has the right to withdraw from the study at any time without being questioned or pressured by anyone. While these guidelines seem to be in favor of the subject, they are. The protection of human rights by institutional review boards consumes much time and, therefore, is costly but serious. Before the advent of such measures, questionable practices were occurring; subjects were coerced and deceived. The ethical treatment of subjects does not seriously jeopardize the research goals of ethical researchers, nor does it bias subjects. It is rare that a person refuses to participate in a project that was presented openly and honestly.

The "exculpatory language" clause has caused researchers in one institution much anguish because the meaning is not obvious. The legal counsels have insisted that it be used as is. The wording is not universal; it is unique to this one institution. Other institutions will have other guidelines. In the absence of any other, the example presented here is acceptable.

Data Collection Methods

The procedure in the example has identified several types of data collection methods. A research method is a way of collecting the data. Such methods include observations, interviews, or questionnaires, and physiological measures. There are many others, but these are basic and provide a good place to begin.

Observation Methods

Observation is something you have been taught almost from your first day in a school of nursing. You have been taught to observe skin color, facial expression, speech patterns, and other behavior. You have been taught to be objective; that is, to separate yourself from the client so that you do not miss or misinterpret important information (data). Those are precisely the skills you use in observing as a method of collecting research data. (Observation skills inherent in nursing make nurses "naturals" as researchers.) You simply must add structure to the process—when, where, and for how long are you going to observe and for what? You need to obtain or compose an observation guide—preferably a checklist because a checklist is the easiest form to use and score.

The checklist may be as simple as checking a "yes" or "no" column depending on whether a behavior (crying, talking) was present or not. The checklist could be more complex with quantities as well. Definitions are needed to clearly describe behavior that will be in a category. "Crying with tears and appearing inconsolable" might be at one end of a continuum, with "whimpering quietly without tears" being at another. Your observation tool will depend on your research question or hypothesis. For a descriptive study, your question might be: What is the distress level of one-year-olds receiving immunization injections in health clinics? You will have defined your variables; your tool will reflect how you define distress; and your observations will be consistent with your definitions, which, of course, are consistent with your conceptual framework.

You must not forget that your presence in any situation will make a difference in the situation. If you go into a clinic to observe, you will possibly alter the behaviors of the clients, parents, and the staff. Children will accommodate your presence faster than adults, because adults are more self-conscious. It is best to have a long enough period for the individuals in the setting to "get used to" your presence before you collect data. If you are participating in the program, it is difficult for you to do two things at once, your job and your research. Try to have someone else relieve you of one.

Interviews

Many beginning researchers are tempted to interview subjects. It sounds so easy. It isn't. If the interview is extremely structured, you might as well have a questionnaire. If the questions of the interview are open ended (cannot be answered with a yes or no or other short answer), the amount of data generated is mammoth and difficult to quantify and interpret. If you use interviewing as your research method, plan to have a limited number of well-chosen subjects (limited because of the impossibility of most beginning researchers to organize and analyze large amounts of data generated by many interviews). Plan for the interview to take much longer than you expect, particularly if it is on a sensitive subject such as death of a significant other. As always, test your interview guide on several individuals and revise the guide as indicated before you begin interviewing subjects. Use a recorder. No, subjects will not be intimidated by the machine. Yes, you must include permission to use it in the subject consent form. Although you will have much work to do in listening to the recordings and scoring them, you will at least have retrievable and, therefore, verifiable data, and you can concentrate on gathering information rather than taking notes during the interview.

Questionnaires

Look at the Exhibit 6-2, Demographic Data Questionnaire. This is a simple tool that was specifically designed for one study. The tool is reasonably clear but could be improved by giving directions at the beginning, rather than repeating "circle one" throughout the questionnaire. The need for the subject's name is not clear; some identifying code that can be matched with other data is more desirable than names. Note that data are clumped together, which will make analysis much simpler than if each subject put exact age. The rationale for gathering the information is given in the procedure. You may or may not agree with the categories, but the subjects should have no trouble understanding what information is being requested.

Standardized questionnaires should provide information about *reliability* and *validity* and the populations on which the tool has been tested. A reliable tool is one that will yield very similar results on the same population at another time and in another situation. Characteristics of a reliable tool include *stability, consistency,* and *equivalence.* Stability, or getting very similar results over time, was indicated for the ANS-IE in the example by the test-retest method and was reported to be $r = 0.83$ over a six-week period. This correlation is considered acceptable by most researchers. Acceptable values vary depending on the situation and the judgment of the researcher, but normally a correlation of 0.70 or higher is considered good enough. Consistency was not addressed for the ANS-IE; consistency refers to all items measuring the same important variable. Also referred to as internal consistency or homogeneity, this quality is measured by comparing the responses on one-half of the tool with the responses on the other half—the split-half method. Other methods for assessing consistency are the Kuder-Richardson formula and Cronbach's alpha. These terms are included here so that you know to what they are referring when you see them in the literature. For further understanding, Polit and Hungler (1983) have a good discussion.

Equivalence has two implications. One is that the tool has equivalent results as other tools known to measure the same variable. The other is that two researchers using the tool would come up with equivalent results. The latter concept of *interrater reliability* is particularly important for observations. Two or more researchers who are going to be making observations must be "trained" and rated; that is, they must observe the same situation at the same time using the tool and compare the results of each researcher's observations for equivalence.

A valid tool is one that measures what it is supposed to measure. A tool cannot be valid if it is not reliable. Types of validity include *face, content, criterion, construct,* and *discriminate.* In the example, discriminate validity is suggested, since the correlation of the ANS-IE with the social desirability scale was 0.10 or 0.06. To state that the ANS-IE scores were not related to the social desirability measure is not quite accurate, since a correlation of 0.00 would be required for there to be no relationship. With the correlation so low, it does appear that the ANS-IE is not measuring social desirability and is, therefore, interpreted as having discriminate validity with regard to social desirability.

Face validity is omitted as a type of validity by some researchers. True, it is not very sophisticated; the only way to evaluate it is to "eyeball" the tool and see if it appears to be asking questions that are getting at what the test is supposed to be designed to do. Still, face validity is useful in some instances. For example, the Demographic Data tool in Exhibit 6-2 appears to have face validity in that the subjects will probably respond with the information the tool is designed to obtain.

Content validity refers to the degree to which the tool covers the content it is designed to measure. Content validity is easiest to understand when considered in the context of classroom testing of content. A good examination will cover proportionately the content of material as it was covered in lecture and textbook and will thus have content validity.

Criterion validity is the establishment of a standard which must be attained in order to make a decision—declare the behavior learned (being accurate 9 times out of 10, making a predetermined score on a paper-and-pencil test, being able to run a mile in 8.5 minutes).

The concepts of interest to researchers are also known as constructs. Anxiety, depression, mothering, nursing care are constructs. There is no way to measure these variables directly, so tools are developed to do so. The degree to which the tools measure the constructs they are designed to measure is construct validity.

There are other criteria for assessing tools; some seem to overlap with validity and reliability; others are common sense. Obviously, a good tool must be an appropriate length for the subjects for whom it is designed. (This may seem obvious, but some enormously long tools have been designed for young children or other individuals who might have short attention spans.) The tool must be worded simply enough and should be sensitive enough to get a spread of scores so that you learn something about your subjects. The data obtained by using the tool should show a difference between the control and the experimental groups (if, indeed, there is a difference).

Physiological Measures

Excerpt 6-1 includes the physiological measure of weight. To be more precise, the researcher might have included the brand of the scale and how calibrated. At least all of the subjects were being weighed on the same scale. Presumably (it should have been clearly stated) the researcher is reading the scale from the same angle for each subject. Similar precautions should be used for all physiological measures—equipment should be as accurate as possible and should be frequently calibrated. Those recording the data should follow the same procedure and be checked for interrater reliability. To be very sure of specimens sent to laboratories, you can send two halves of the same sample and compare the reports of each. Set up an organized system for recording the data so that you are assured of accuracy.

Potential Error Sources

Errors will still occur even with the best of tools. The best way to keep errors to a minimum is to be aware of potential sources and take precautions to prevent them. Errors may occur due to environmental factors—too hot, too cold, too noisy, anything that might be distracting. The time of day may vary from one administration of the tool to another, so that subjects may be variously hungry, tired, angry, or disinterested. The researcher may have a different effect on various subjects. Some subjects tend to respond the way they perceive the researcher wants them to respond; others may be antagonistic and respond the opposite of what they believe is desirable. Every effort should be made to make the subjects comfortable and administer tools in the best environment possible.

The Research Proposal

The research proposal includes all of the steps in the research process that have been presented. Research committees vary as to how much detail is required about the review of the literature and the conceptual framework. Hypotheses and/or research questions are imperative; so is a detailed procedure, with the research method clearly presented and any research tools included or clearly described.

FOLLOWING THE PLAN

The best laid plans often go astray and research is no exception. Be careful. Interpersonal relationships with individuals who are in positions to facilitate or obstruct the collection of your data are most important. If you "sell" your idea to the head nurses of the units where you would like to collect data you will have a much easier job than if you ignore or offend someone. Spending a little time explaining what you are doing and why will pay great dividends later.

When the process does not go as planned, in spite of all you can do, go back to your research committee or adviser. Believe it or not, these sources are intended to be helpful, not just obstructive. They have had more experience and know how to facilitate your problem solving. Rarely is it necessary to abandon an idea completely and start over. Some aspect of the problem is usually salvageable.

Some of the calamities that befall the researcher include the unforeseeable decrease in the number of potential subjects meeting the research criteria: no hysterectomies done during the months you planned to see if a liquid diet 24 hours before surgery would decrease the intensity of postoperative gas pains; a new group of psychiatric residents tend to diagnose patients as having adjustment reaction when you had planned to study the effects of long term assignment of nurses to individuals newly diagnosed as having schizophrenia; or mothers of newborns begin going home 48 hours after giving birth so that you cannot observe mother-infant interactions on days 3 and 4. Obviously, the way to try to prevent such disappointments is to know as much as possible about your potential study population before you plan your procedure.

SUMMARY

Collecting research data logically follows the identification of a problem; the review of the literature; the placing of the problem within a conceptual framework; identification and definition of the variables; choice of a research method that fits the research question or hypothesis; and the choice of a reliable and valid research tool to be administered according to a carefully elaborated procedure. All of these steps are put together into a paper called a research proposal that must be approved by the appropriate committees before the data can be collected.

Chapter 7 includes discussion of what to do with the data after you get them.

Suggestions for Further Study

In order to gain some experience with the ideas presented in this chapter, the following exercises are suggested:

1. In some of the research articles you have already read (or choose new ones), find the research methods used to collect the data.

2. Find three research articles that include a discussion of research tools used. How were the reliability and validity assessed?

3. In a study group, assign each person to weigh at home before coming to the next class and bring that weight on a piece of paper to the next class. At the next class have a scale and have each person weigh. Compare the results of the two weights. What are probable sources of error for any differences?

4. Write a procedure including method for the research problem you have been working on. Discuss it with peers and faculty. What are the strengths of the procedure? What could be improved?

5. Assign a research article for each person in your discussion group to read and prepare a detailed discussion of how each of you believes the research was conducted. Was there sufficient information for the study to be replicated?

Suggestions for Additional Reading

Brink, P. J., and Wood, M. J. *Basic Steps in Planning Nursing Research* (2nd edition). Monterey, CA: Wadsworth Health Sciences Division, 1983. (Chapters 8 and 9)

Buros, O. (Ed.). *The Eighth Mental Measurement Yearbook.* Hyland Park, NJ: Gryphon Press, 1978.

Fox, D. J. *Fundamentals of Research in Nursing* (4th edition). Norwalk, CN: Appleton-Century-Crofts, 1982. (Chapters 13–17)

Kerlinger, F. N. *Foundations of Behavioral Research.* New York: Holt, Rinehart and Winston, Inc., 1964.

Polit, D. F., and Hungler, B. P. *Nursing Research: Principles and Methods* (2nd edition). Philadelphia: J. B. Lippincott Company, 1983. (Chapters 12–16)

Seaman, C. H., and Verhonick, P. J. *Research Methods for Undergraduate Students in Nursing* (2nd edition). New York: Appleton-Century-Crofts, 1982. (Chapters 10–12)

White, C. M., and Ruth, M. V. "Data Collection: Data-Generating Instruments" in S. D. Krampitz and N. Pavlovich (Eds.), *Readings for Nursing Research.* St. Louis: The C. V. Mosby Company, 1981.

Chapter 7
What are you going to do with it when you get it?

ORGANIZATION AND ANALYSIS OF DATA

Chapter Objectives

> Upon successful completion of this chapter, the student will be able to

- Differentiate among the concepts of descriptive, inferential, and correlational statistics
- Describe the advantages of using computers in data analysis
- Classify data according to nominal, ordinal, interval, and ratio scales
- Differentiate between parametric and nonparametric tests
- Compute selected measures of central tendency, variability, correlation, and inferential statistics
- Define the terms homogeneity of variance and normal distribution
- Define null hypothesis
- Make appropriate decisions of accepting or rejecting the null hypothesis

INTRODUCTION

The purpose of all that you have been through is to communicate with others, particularly the nursing community. That is, you have identified a problem, put the problem into a conceptual framework, reviewed what others have done about the same or similar problems, designed a study to add to what is already known, and collected data according to your design. Now that you have all of these figures, or examples, or tabulations, you must *organize* the data in such a way that you have evidence for making a statement about the original problem of concern (which may seem quite remote after all you have done). In addition to organizing the data, you will want (or you will be urged) to *analyze* the data in such a way that your statement will have some weight if the data have a different probability than would be expected by chance.

You might think of the data collection as similar to grocery shopping. You carefully identify what your needs are, make a list as indicated, and go to the appropriate supermarket to purchase the items on your list. While this procedure may be relatively automatic for you, the process is well defined and the steps to the goal of replenishing your bare cupboards are deliberately executed. Your collection of the items into your shopping cart is not haphazard; you collect the items according to the way the store has them arranged—probably aisle by aisle. If you are a fairly organized individual you may have made out your list according to your mental image of the arrangement of the items in the market. (Your plan for data collection should have been no less precise.) At any rate, you proceed to collect the desired items. It is quite likely that you will not get exactly what you planned because supermarkets are sometimes out of certain items, packaging is changed, and prices increase. In spite of the difficulties encountered, you stick to your plan as carefully as possible. Thus you have your "collection."

When you get home and unload your car, all of your groceries will be in bags—hidden from your view and unorganized. In that state, your groceries are not useful. You must unbag the items and place them in appropriate places. Some of the items will be processed further at a later time, others will be used after merely being washed (cleaned up). Some items require more sorting and preparation for storage than others. In addition, the more organizing and treatment you do at the time of storage, the less attention you will need to give the items later. Needless to say you make sure that nothing gets lost. (Some of this analogy can be taken literally, as individuals have been known to store their theses or dissertations in the vegetable tray of the refrigerator because, if the building burns, that container is the least likely to be destroyed. Don't laugh—once you have gotten this far you have become *very* attached to your data.)

When you are ready to use the stored items, you must retrieve them from the cupboards, refrigerator, or freezer. Some items will be ready for use (eating) just as they are; for example, fruits and vegetables may be eaten raw. Even with these items, it will be necessary to "clean them up," manipulate them so that they are consumable (peel them, cut or break them up), and arrange them so that the consumer is enticed to internalize them (or eat them).

So it is with data. They must be cleaned up to be made readable and accurate (uncontaminated). Data must be manipulated to be consumable. Placed in tables or displayed in figures, data may be made more palpable and easier to "swallow," understand, or internalize.

Other items you purchased at the store will require more preparation to be edible. Even if the items could be consumed without the elaborate preparation, they would not be as interesting (meaningful). Such preparation may include cooking, baking, marinating, or more elaborate treatment. Obviously, what you do to the food depends on the nature of the food item and your goal. Likewise, a collection of numbers has some meaning if presented "raw" but may take on more importance if "treated" in certain ways. The treatment depends on the nature of the data and on the message you wish to convey. Neither the nature of the data nor the message can be considered independent of the other.

Fruit in a fruit bowl, arranged attractively for display and consumption, is similar to descriptive data in tables or figures for visual consumption of information. Simple preparation, such as toasting or warming food, is not unlike simple manipulations of data in obtaining percentages and measurements of central tendency. (In other words, what you see is what you get.)

As you prepare food in more elaborate ways, the outcome hardly resembles what you began with. A cake or a souffle bears little resemblance to the eggs, milk, and flour that went into the pan to be cooked, where the ingredients were transformed into something quite different and much more delicious. So data may be put into a computer (or even manipulated by a hand calculator), and the output may not resemble the input.

When we infer something more than the literal output of the data, we are using *inferential statistics* rather than the *descriptive statistics* used when we were just rearranging the numbers for better display. With inferential statistics, we infer that something did or did not happen as a result of *chance*. Chance means that certain things are going to happen in spite of our input (or intervention). We know, for example, that of a group of individuals diagnosed as having an emotional problem, one-third of them will get better with or without treatment, one-third of them will get better with treatment, and one-third of them will not get better no matter what. Therefore, if you provided treatment and clients got better, how do you know if your treatment made the difference or if you were merely treating the ones who were going to improve anyway? You would use inferential statistics to determine (within a predetermined level of probability) if your data might have occurred by chance alone or if the data you generated were outside the scope of a chance happening. (You will encounter other definitions of inferential statistics; the one presented here is elementary and included for understanding—not for sophistication.)

While we are classifying statistics, let's complete the set. *Correlation* techniques are frequently used in data collected by nurses because we frequently ask such questions as: Is an increase in a certain treatment associated with an increase in activity (defined as healthy)? In other words, if one variable increases, does the other one increase? In this case, we are examining a relationship. The answer to the question is a number between -1.0 and $+1.0$. A correlation of -1.0 means that as one variable increases the other always decreases; a correlation of $+1.0$ means that as one variable increases the other variable always increases; and a correlation of 0.0 means there is no relationship. The correlation is a description of the degree of the relationship, it does not infer whether the correlation is a chance occurrence or not. Additional statistical tests must be done in order to make any inferences. The techniques for making inferences will be described and illustrated later in this chapter. The important point here is that once you have determined a correlation, you still do not have a probability until further tests have been performed.

There are some advanced statistical techniques that will not be dealt with in this book because they might be considered "gourmet" types and are outside the capabilities of most individuals who do not possess access to a computer. In fact, multiple regression, for example, was rarely used until the computer became available. The reason is obviously that the mathematical manipulations are so extensive that to perform the indicated operations by hand is prohibitive. The same reasoning is true of complex analyses of variance (anything beyond a simple one-way analysis). While these manipulations might possibly be done by hand, it makes no more sense to do so than to rub two sticks together to build a fire to cook a gourmet meal. Except under unusual circumstances, it makes more sense to buy a match and use conventional equipment. If you do not have access to a computer and statistical consultation, it is as unlikely that you will be able to perform an analysis of variance (ANOVA) or multiple regressions as for you to produce a recognizable Beef Wellington over an outdoor wood fire. Therefore, this book will neither provide formulas for multiple regressions and ANOVAs nor recipes for Beef Wellington. If you do not have the knowledge and equipment for gourmet cooking yet, eat more simply until you acquire them. If you do not have the knowledge and resources for using advanced statistics, design simpler studies until you can obtain the necessary skills and equipment.

All of the statistical tests presented in this chapter were computed with a hand calculator and are within the capabilities of anyone who can accurately calculate drug dosages. Formulas are deliberately omitted so that the presentations are in "English" and can be read and followed by any literate individual. There are numerous ways of calculating many of the tests. Many have slightly different methods depending on the number of cases, whether pairs are matched, and other variables. The tests are merely examples of the most frequently used and most useful of the tests.

COMPUTERS

We are living in the age of the computer. Our children are going to be much more sophisticated than we because they are growing up with these machines. Sixth graders are doing reports on word processors; adolescents are spending many quarters at neighborhood video game rooms; adults are trying to figure out how they can make the computer manipulate their finances in order to justify a generous income tax refund.

The computer is no less important for the researcher. The modern serious researcher would enhance his or her research capabilities immeasurably by negotiating access to computer usage and developing computer literacy. The primary advantages of computers are accuracy and speed. Those qualities make it possible for the computer to perform lengthy and complex operations. Using a computer is no more complicated than using an electric typewriter—you simply follow a set of instructions. The instructions vary considerably, from the microcomputers to the institutional ones, and depend somewhat on how the user is billed for the cost of using the computer. Another variable is whether you would get the output (printout of your work) at the terminal (point where you put it in) or whether you would have to pick up the printout elsewhere.

Since the variables associated with obtaining access to and using a computer are numerous, any specific instructions given here would have to be modified considerably for each individual. My suggestion is that you avail yourself of any and every opportunity to learn about and gain access to computers for the purpose of using them for your research. (You will not learn very much about research by playing any of the numerous computer games—but you might have fun.) Do not be afraid to ask questions no matter how stupid they may seem to you. Our children may grow up with sophisticated knowledge about computers, but we are going to have to learn about the computers through adult education.

TYPES OF DATA

All numbers do not have the same meaning. Just as some foods are liquids and some are solids, and you treat solids differently from the way you treat liquids (you serve juice in a glass rather than on a napkin), you treat some numbers differently from the way you treat others. Numbers are classified according to what they measure. They may also be called scales or rules (meaning graduated). Numbers are broadly classified as nonmetric or metric measurements (Brogan 1981). Nonmetric scales may be subdivided into nominal and ordinal measurements; metric scales are subdivided into interval and ratio measurements.

1. Nonmetric measurements
   a) Nominal
   b) Ordinal
2. Metric measurements
   a) Interval
   b) Ratio

Nominal

Nominal measurements merely name. They represent a shorthand for putting items into categories. The forms you complete to renew your membership in the American Nurses' Association represent nominal categories. There is no numerical difference between the category "male" and that of "female," even though one may be labeled "1" and the other "2." Likewise, there are no numerical differences between the categories "married," "single," "divorced," or "widowed," in spite of the assignment of numbers 1–4 to those groups. With this type of data, you can report *frequencies* referring to the number of individuals in each category. You could determine the ratio of men to women or married to single. You could report what percentage each group is of the entire membership. Nominal data are also referred to as categorical data, frequency data, attribute data, or enumeration data (Edwards 1958).

Ordinal

Ordinal scales imply a hierarchy in the order. Members of the set logically come before or after some other members. Think of Erikson's (1963) eight stages of development: there is order; one stage logically comes before another, but they are by no means equal. The stage of trust versus mistrust is usually considerably shorter than the stage of generativity versus stagnation. There are exceptions, as in the case of developmentally delayed individuals who may experience a very lengthy trust versus mistrust stage and a brief generativity versus stagnation stage; if in fact, they reach the generativity stage at all. Nevertheless, the stages occur in order: trust versus mistrust; autonomy versus shame and doubt; initiative versus guilt; industry versus inferiority; identity versus role diffusion; intimacy versus isolation; generativity versus stagnation; and ego integrity versus despair.

Another example of an ordinal scale is that of a map that is not drawn to scale. The landmarks along the routes are listed, but the distances between the places vary. You would pass them in order, but you could not measure the distance between any two points to determine how far it is from the beginning to the end of the journey. A type of ordinal scale used frequently in nursing research is a "Likert"-type scale, which ranks responses in some order such as "very frequently," "frequently," "sometimes," "seldom," and "almost never." Ordinal scales are also referred to as ranks.

Interval

Interval scales have equal and measurable differences between segments. The best example of an interval scale is the thermometer. The difference between 98 degrees Farenheit and 99 degrees Farenheit is the same as the difference between 98 degrees and 97 degrees. It is inappropriate to say that an increase in temperature of one degree is a one percent increase because there is no base zero. Zero on the thermometer is an arbitrary point.

Ratio

Ratio scales have equal intervals and a meaningful zero point. Height and weight are ratio measurements. A child who is four feet tall is twice as tall as a child who is two feet tall. Likewise, an individual who weighs 120 pounds is three times as heavy as one who weighs 40 pounds (however useful that information may be). Distances between two points are ratio data. Given that your car consumes a steady amount of gasoline, you must have twice as much gas to travel 200 miles as 100 miles.

Why do you need this information? You need to know the nature of your data in order to analyze it appropriately. In a "Peanuts" cartoon (Schulz 1976), Marcie was trying to learn how to dye Easter eggs. Peppermint Patty told her to *cook* the eggs. She did—over light. After obtaining more eggs, Peppermint Patty told Marcie not to fry them this time. Marcie proceeded to put them successively in the toaster, the oven, and the waffle iron. "No!" Peppermint Patty finally screamed, "Boil them!" Marcie did—after cracking them. The result was egg soup (and no colored Easter eggs). The point is that unless you have some idea of the end product you are expecting, you may treat your data inappropriately (and the result could be worse than egg soup).

Another (and perhaps somewhat more relevant) example is the nature of scores on intelligence tests. IQ scores are, at most, interval scales; but are they really that exact or are they ordinal? Is the difference between a person with an IQ of 100 and one with an IQ of 130 the same as the difference between that same person with 100 IQ and a person with an IQ of 70? Arguments have been posed both ways. The point is that you should be aware of the type of data you are collecting and analyzing.

The importance of understanding the rules associated with the measurement scales will become more apparent to you in future discussions. At this point, you simply need to be aware that you can do some things with some kinds of data that you cannot do (reasonably) with others. For example, in order to determine which house in the neighborhood is the most representative of the lifestyle in that community, you would not add all of the house numbers and divide by the number of houses in order to get an "average," even though the numbers on a given street are ranked so that you would expect 1349 to appear before 1353, which would be before 1367. Also, if you know the range of the numbers on a given street, you could estimate the relative position of the house you are seeking. In that sense, the "average" number on that street might be the house close to the middle of the street. It does not give you any information about the quality of the house.

Equally ludicrous is the idea of determining the best ball player by choosing the one with the highest number on the jersey. (Whether or not you can choose the best automobile by picking the one with the highest sticker price is debatable.) When you begin to think of making some inferences from your data, you will get more experience in applying the rules and understanding which data are appropriate for which tests; and, conversely, which tests are based on certain assumptions about the nature of the data collected. Tables 7-1 through 7-4 provide summaries of the types of measurement scales, examples, and appropriate mathematical manipulations as well as some inferential types of tests that can be applied.

TABLE 7-1
Measures of Central Tendency according to Types of Scale

TYPE OF SCALE	MEASURE OF CENTRAL TENDENCY
Nominal	Mode
	Frequency
Ordinal	Median
	Percentile
Interval	Mean
Ratio	Mean

TABLE 7-2
Measures of Variability according to Types of Scale

TYPE OF SCALE	MEASURE OF VARIABILITY (DISPERSION)
Nominal	(None logical)
Ordinal	Range
	Interquartile range
	Semi-interquartile range
Interval	Standard deviation
	Variance
Ratio	Standard deviation
	Variance

TABLE 7-3
Tests of Correlation according to Types of Scale

TYPE OF SCALE	TEST OF CORRELATION
Nominal	Contingency coefficient
Ordinal	Spearman rho
	Kendall's Tau
	Kendall W
Interval	Pearson product moment correlation
	Multiple product moment correlation
Ratio	Pearson product moment correlation
	Multiple product moment correlation

TABLE 7-4
Inferential Statistics according to Type of Scale

TYPE OF SCALE	INFERENTIAL STATISTICS
Nominal	Chi square
	Binomial
	McNamar test for the significance of changes
	Fisher exact probability test
	Cochran Q test
Ordinal	Kolmogorov-Smirnov test
	Runs test
	Sign test
	Wilcoxon matched pairs signed rank test
	Median test
	Mann Whitney-U
	Friedman 2-way ANOVA
	Kruskal-Wallis one-way ANOVA
Interval	t-test
	ANOVA
Ratio	t-test
	ANOVA

Two points you need to know about the statistical concepts represented in Tables 7-1 through 7-4 are

1. The operations or tests appropriate for each type of scale include all of the operations or tests indicated for each lower order scale. For example, although the median is indicated as the appropriate measure of central tendency for the ordinal type of data, it is acceptable to report the mode or frequency for ordinal data. Likewise, although the t-test is indicated as the appropriate inferential test for interval data, it is acceptable to do a Mann-Whitney U test on interval data. It is not permissible to go in the opposite direction. You may not (logically) report means for nominal data.

2. The tests indicated for nonmetric (nominal and ordinal data) are known as nonparametric statistical tests in contrast to the tests indicated for metric data (interval and ratio), which are referred to as parametric statistical tests. Nonparametric inferential tests are used on

any data (nonmetric or metric) when the following basic assumptions cannot be met: random sampling, normal distribution, and homogeneity of variance. The concept of random sampling is familiar to you from the discussion in Chapter 5 on selection of subjects. Normal distribution will be included in the discussion below of measures of central tendency. Homogeneity of variance will be included later in this chapter in the discussion of inferential parametric statistics.

DESCRIPTIVE STATISTICS

As suggested earlier, descriptive statistics describe. That is, descriptive statistics are used to present the data in such a way as to be meaningful and create a picture of the information obtained. Two types of descriptive data are measures of central tendency and measures of variability.

Measures of Central Tendency

As illustrated in Table 7-1, measures of central tendency include frequency, mode, median, mean, and percentile. These terms are used to describe variables and are, therefore, useful descriptive statistics. Runyon-Haber (1971) defined a measure of central tendency as "an index of central location employed in the description of frequency distributions" (p. 56). What do the data look like? Where are the most frequently occurring points? First, we will discuss frequency distributions, followed by discussions and examples of modes, medians, and means. The term "average" as used by the lay public is confusing because it may refer to either the mode, median, or mean and have different implications depending on how the "average" is derived.

Frequency simply means how many and is determined by counting. The number of men and the number of women in a given geographic location are frequencies. The number of individuals in various age categories is the frequency. Note that we are referring to nominal data and are counting the number of items in a category. You will quickly reach a point with frequency data where the information is too cumbersome to be meaningful. Suppose you are reporting the number of items correctly answered by each of 100 students on a 100-question physiology examination. Information in such detail is more than most persons want to know. Therefore, you organize your data into a frequency distribution, from students who missed the least number of items to those who missed the most.

For further illustration, consider grades on an examination. The grades for 100 students might appear as follows:

47	98	67	32	78	92	55	77	89	63
69	87	71	88	61	93	48	84	97	82
87	96	96	69	96	89	87	39	97	76
99	30	87	41	55	79	75	92	54	47
99	59	79	40	98	69	52	53	66	65
88	62	48	62	93	94	55	87	63	50
65	42	84	94	87	55	72	87	94	66
91	50	60	63	60	94	73	56	86	64
80	58	60	99	64	59	79	78	66	91
67	76	55	89	62	43	99	85	63	54

Looking at this array of numbers does not give you much information. Some would even describe this jumble as overwhelming. To organize these numbers into a frequency distribution, in order to make them more meaningful, you would arrange them in order from the highest score to the lowest and note how many of each score occurred—that is, the frequency of each score. You should derive the following distribution:

SCORE (X)	FREQUENCY (f)	SCORE (X)	FREQUENCY (f)
99	4	67	2
98	2	66	3
97	2	65	2
96	3	64	2
94	4	63	4
93	2	62	3
92	2	61	1
91	2	60	3
89	3	59	2
88	2	58	1
87	7	56	1
86	1	55	5
85	1	54	2
84	2	53	1
82	1	52	1
80	1	50	2
79	3	48	2
78	2	47	2

SCORE (X)	FREQUENCY (f)	SCORE (X)	FREQUENCY (f)
77	1	43	1
76	2	42	1
75	1	41	1
73	1	40	1
72	1	39	1
71	1	32	1
69	3	30	1

Note on the frequency distribution table the scores that did not occur are not listed; for example, 31, 33, 34, 35, 36, 37, 38, 44, and others do not appear on the table because no one made those grades. In this group of 100 scores the percentage of occurrence is the same as the frequency; that is, four of the students made 99 on the examination and that was 4 percent of the students.

Another way of organizing these data is to group the scores at equal intervals; for example, if you grouped the scores in intervals of 5 you would obtain the following distribution:

SCORES (X)	FREQUENCY (f)	CUMULATIVE FREQUENCY (cf)
99–95	11	100
94–90	10	89
89–85	14	79
84–80	4	65
79–75	9	61
74–70	3	52
69–65	10	49
64–60	13	39
59–55	9	26
54–50	6	17
49–45	4	11
44–40	4	7
39–35	1	3
34–30	2	2

The *mode* is the most frequently occurring value (in this case, grade). With the data as we have organized it so far, we could report the mode in one of two ways: as the most frequently occurring individual score (87, since that was the score made by seven students and no other score was made by so many students) or as the most frequently occurring interval of scores (89–85, since that was the interval of scores made by 14 students). In this example, the two ways of reporting the mode include the same scores, but it is possible for the interval mode to occur at different points than the individual score mode.

The *median* is the "middle" score, or the score above which half of the students scored (and below which the other half scored). Looking at our interval distribution, it is easy to see that half of these scores are in and above the 74–70 interval. For most purposes that is as close as we would want to know. We could, however, look on the individual frequency scores table to see the exact score that is the dividing point. It turns out that 50 students scored 72 and above and 50 scored 71 and below. If pressed to identify an arithmetic median we would have to split the difference and indicate 71.5.

Percentiles are used in communicating to individuals how they compare with others who took the same test. If one is in the 75th percentile, that individual made a score as high or higher than 75 percent of the others taking the test. In our example, the individuals making 85 and above are in the 75th percentile.

The *mean* or average may be logically determined in the example given because the scores are interval. In other words, there is the same numerical difference between 77 and 78 as there is between 78 and 79, if we obtained the score from the number of problems answered according to the answer key. (If we try to imply something about how much information an individual has acquired based on these scores, we could have difficulty. For example, does the person who made 82 really know twice as much as the one who made 41? Probably not, but the person who made 82 did answer twice as many questions correctly as did the person who made 41. Be clear about what you are reporting.) The mean is obtained by adding each of the grades and dividing by the total number of grades. In the example, the average is 72.21. Note the difference between this average and the mode of 87 as indicated earlier. Think about what is generally implied by the average grade (that it is about the norm) and what these figures indicate (that the implication changes depending on which statistic you report). The mean in the example is very close to the median of 71.5.

Measures of Variability

Another way of describing data is by reporting *measures of variability* (also known as *dispersion*). For any data (except nominal) you could report the *range*, which is simply the lowest and the highest values obtained. In the example we have been considering, the range of scores is from 30 to 99, or

69. Range can be reported in interquartiles, which is defined as the range of scores between the 75th and the 25th quartiles (84 to 55, or 29 in our example). Semi-interquartile range is, as the term implies, half the distance between the 75th and the 25th quartiles, or half of 29, or 14.5.

The *standard deviation* is the average of the deviation of scores from the mean. The standard deviation is a useful and frequently reported statistic. The following steps will be useful in computing the standard deviation of a set of scores:

1. Add up each of the scores (obtain the sum).
2. Divide the sum by the number of scores (obtain the mean).
3. Subtract the mean from each score.
4. Square each of the values obtained in step 3.
5. Add up all of the squares from step 4 (obtain the sum of squares).
6. Divide the sum of squares by the number of scores. This figure is the variance.
7. Obtain the square root of the variance. The square root of the variance is the standard deviation.

To illustrate these seven steps, let's go to a new example because the grades used in previous examples are too cumbersome for easy computations. Suppose you wanted to know the standard deviation of the lengths of newborns (rounded off to whole inches) of mothers who were on a food supplement program during the second and third trimesters of pregnancy. The ten infants in the study were 18, 19, 19, 19, 21, 19, 20, 22, 23, and 20 inches long.

X Means	Difference	Square of Difference
$18 - 20$	$= -2 \, (\times -2)$	$= 4$
$19 - 20$	$= -1 \, (\times -1)$	$= 1$
$19 - 20$	$= -1 \, (\times -1)$	$= 1$
$19 - 20$	$= -1 \, (\times -1)$	$= 1$
$19 - 20$	$= -1 \, (\times -1)$	$= 1$
$20 - 20$	$= 0 \, (\times \ 0)$	$= 0$
$20 - 20$	$= 0 \, (\times \ 0)$	$= 0$
$21 - 20$	$= 1 \, (\times \ 1)$	$= 1$
$22 - 20$	$= 2 \, (\times \ 2)$	$= 4$
$23 - 20$	$= 3 \, (\times \ 3)$	$= \underline{9}$
Sum $= 200 \div 10$	$= 20$ (mean)	22 = Sum of Squares

The sum of the lengths divided by the number of infants is 20 (the average or mean length). The sum of the squares of the differences of the mean from each length is 22. Twenty-two divided by the number of infants (10) is 2.2, the variance. The square root of 2.2 is 1.48, the standard deviation. (Square roots of whole numbers from 1 to 100 are given in Appendix E. Most hand calculators now have the square root function, which simplifies calculating square roots of numbers containing decimals.)

Standard deviations are most useful in populations which are assumed to be normally distributed. A *normal distribution* is a distribution in which the values (if all were known) would fall in a bell-shaped curve. That is, very few values would be at either extreme and the frequency of occurrence would increase as you approach the middle of the continuum. In a normal distribution, the median, mean, and mode coincide. One standard deviation on either side of the mean in a normal distribution contains 34.13 percent of the population. The sum of one standard deviation above and one standard deviation below the mean is 68.26 percent of the population. The further you go toward either extreme, the fewer members of the population will be represented. Between one and two standard deviations above the mean 13.59 percent of the population will be found. The same proportion will fall between one and two standard deviations below the mean. Less than 5 percent of a normally distributed population falls outside two standard deviations on either side of the mean.

Many naturally occurring phenomena are normally distributed. Heights, weights, IQs, income tend to fall along a bell-shaped curve. In the study of the lengths of infants, if there were a very large number and if the lengths were normally distributed, 68.26 percent of the newborns would be between 21.48 and 18.52 inches long, and 95.4 percent would be between 22.96 and 17.04 inches.

TESTS OF CORRELATION

As mentioned earlier in this chapter, correlations test relationships between variables. Depending on the type of scale the data represent (nominal, ordinal, interval, or ratio) the appropriate correlation test would be contingency coefficient (for nominal data), Spearman rho (for ordinal data), or Pearson product moment correlation (for interval and ratio data).

Contingency Coefficient Correlation

The *contingency coefficient correlation* is appropriate for answering such questions as what is the relationship between the region of the country in which one lives and the basic nursing program from which one graduated? To determine such a relationship, set up a table showing the distribution of the data collected. (No assumptions about random sampling or normal distribution are required.)

TABLE 7-5
Observed Frequencies of Graduation from Basic Nursing Programs in Regions of the Country (fictitious data)

PROGRAM TYPE	NE	SE	NC	SC	NW	SW	TOTALS
Diploma	20	10	5	5	5	5	50
Associate Degree	40	10	5	5	5	5	70
Baccalaureate	20	10	10	5	10	5	60
Generic Master's	12	2	1	1	1	3	20
Totals	92	32	21	16	21	18	200

First we compute the *chi square value* for these data. To do so, proceed according to the following steps:

1. Determine the *expected* value of each cell. The intersect of each region and program is a cell. (In the cell indicating the number of diploma graduates living in the northeast, the value is 20.) The expected value is determined for each cell by multiplying the marginal totals and dividing by the total number of subjects. For the diploma/northeast cell, the expected value is $92 \times 50 \div 200 = 23$, as indicated in Table 7-6. The expected value in each cell is indicated in the respective cell. The values in the cells in Table 7-5 are *observed* values; the values in the cells in Table 7-6 are the *expected* values.

TABLE 7-6
Expected Frequencies of Graduation from Basic Nursing Programs in Regions of the Country

PROGRAM TYPE	NE	SE	NC	SC	NW	SW	TOTALS
Diploma	23	8	5.25	4	5.25	4.5	50
Associate Degree	32.2	11.2	7.35	5.6	7.35	6.3	70
Baccalaureate	27.6	9.6	6.3	4.8	6.3	5.4	60
Generic Master's	9.2	3.2	2.1	1.6	2.1	1.8	20
Totals	92	32	21	16	21	18	200

2. Subtract the expected value from the observed value (to get the *difference*); square the difference (to get the *product*). Divide the product by the expected value. In the example, your calculations should yield the results shown in Table 7-7.

TABLE 7-7. Calculations of Chi Square (χ^2)

$(20 - 23)^2/23 =$	$9/23 =$	.39
$(10 - 8)^2/8 =$	$4/8 =$	.50
$(5 - 5.25)^2/5.25 =$	$.0625/5.25 =$	.01
$(5 - 4)^2/4 =$	$1/4 =$	.25
$(5 - 5.25)^2/5.25 =$	$.0625/5.25 =$	.01
$(5 - 4.5)^2/4.5 =$	$.25/4.5 =$	.06
$(40 - 32.2)^2/32.2 =$	$60.84/32.2 =$	1.89
$(10 - 11.2)^2/11.2 =$	$1.44/11.2 =$	.13
$(5 - 7.35)^2/7.35 =$	$5.52/7.35 =$	.75
$(5 - 5.6)^2/5.6 =$	$.36/5.6 =$	.06
$(5 - 7.35)^2/7.35 =$	$5.52/7.35 =$	.75
$(5 - 6.3)^2/6.3 =$	$1.69/6.3 =$	.27
$(20 - 27.6)^2/27.6 =$	$57.76/27.6 =$	2.09
$(10 - 9.6)^2/9.6 =$	$.16/9.6 =$	.02
$(10 - 6.3)^2/6.3 =$	$13.69/6.3 =$	2.17
$(5 - 4.8)^2/4.8 =$	$.04/4.8 =$	.01
$(10 - 6.3)^2/6.3 =$	$13.69/6.3 =$	2.17
$(5 - 5.4)^2/5.4 =$	$.16/5.4 =$	.03
$(12 - 9.2)^2/9.2 =$	$7.84/9.2 =$	.85
$(2 - 3.2)^2/3.2 =$	$1.44/3.2 =$	.45
$(1 - 2.1)^2/2.1 =$	$1.21/2.1 =$	.58
$(1 - 1.6)^2/1.6 =$	$.36/1.6 =$	.23
$(1 - 2.1)^2/2.1 =$	$1.21/2.1 =$	.58
$(3 - 1.8)^2/1.8 =$	$1.44/1.8 =$	.80
	Sum $=$	15.05

3. Add the quotients to obtain the chi square (χ^2) value, which in this example is 15.05.

Now that we have the chi square value, we can compute the contingency coefficient of our sample. The steps are

1. Divide chi square (15.05) by the number of subjects in the sample (200) plus chi square (15.05).

$$15.05/(200 + 15.05) = .07$$

2. Find the square root of the results in step 1 (.07). In this example the square root of .07 is .26. The contingency coefficient in this example is .26.

The relationship between the region of the country in which one lives and the type of nursing program from which one graduated is not a strong one in our example. The closer the correlation is to 1 (or −1), the stronger the relationship.

Spearman rho Correlation

The *Spearman rho correlation* requires that both variables be measured in at least an ordinal scale so that the data can be ranked in two ordered series. Data to answer the question "What is the relationship between attitudes toward elderly and socioeconomic status (SES)?" could be analyzed with a Spearman rho correlation. For example, assume the scores of the attitudes scale have a possible range of 1 to 25, with 1 being the least favorable attitude and 25 being the most favorable. The SES include low-low, middle-low, high-low, low-middle, middle-middle, high-middle, low-high, middle-high, and high-high. For 10 individuals, the data in Table 7-8 might be obtained.

TABLE 7-8
Hypothetical Example of Spearman rho Correlation Coefficient

SUBJECT	SCORE	RANK	SES	RANK	DIFFERENCE	D^2
A	19	(10)	low-low	(1)	9	81
B	5	(4)	high-middle	(7)	−3	9
C	8	(6)	low-middle	(5)	1	1
D	14	(8)	high-low	(3.5)	4.5	20.25
E	2	(1)	high-high	(10)	−9	81
F	6	(5)	middle-middle	(6)	−1	1
G	15	(9)	middle-low	(2)	7	49
H	3	(2)	high-low	(3.5)	−1.5	2.25
I	4	(3)	low-high	(8)	−5	25
J	10	(7)	middle-high	(9)	−2	4
				Sums	0	273.5

To compute the Spearman rho correlation

1. Rank each subject on both variables as indicated in the parentheses in Table 7-8. Note that for a tie the *average* of the rankings, had they not been tied, is assigned to each subject in the tie. (Technically, if the

proportion of ties is "large," a correction factor should be used. See Siegel, 1956. For a minimal number of ties, the effect of ties is negligible.)

2. Obtain the *difference* between the ranks for each subject as indicated in the "Difference" column in Table 7-8. Note that the sum of the difference should equal zero (0).

3. Square the differences, as in the D^2 column, and obtain the sum of the squares (273.5 in the example).

4. Multiply 6 (a fixed number derived for computation—will be used no matter what your data are) by the sum of the squares ($6 \times 273.5 =$ 1641).

5. Divide the figure obtained in step 4 by the cube of the number of subjects minus the number of subjects. In the example, the number of subjects is 10; 10 cubed is $10 \times 10 \times 10$, or 1000.

$$1000 - 10 = 990$$
$$1641/990 = 1.66$$

6. Subtract the figure obtained in 5 from 1.

$$1 - 1.66 = -.66$$

The Spearman rho in this example is $-.66$. The minus indicates there is a *negative* correlation. In our fictitious example, the interpretation of the data might be that as the socioeconomic status increases, the attitudes toward the elderly decrease (are less positive).

Pearson Product Moment Correlation

The *Pearson product moment correlation,* or *Pearson r,* is the appropriate correlation statistic for interval and ratio data. Data such as age, weight, and height are data to which the Pearson *r* may be applied. For a simple example, suppose we wanted to determine the relationship of weight and height of a group of 16-year-old males who weighed 170, 140, 120, 180, and 200 pounds. The respective heights are 72, 66, 64, 72, and 73 inches. To calculate the Pearson *r* using the raw score method (Runyon-Haber 1971), make the table shown in Table 7-9.

Obtain the standard deviation of X as follows:

$$\sqrt{\frac{135300}{5} - (162)^2} = \sqrt{27,060 - 26,244} = \sqrt{816} = 28.57$$

Obtain the standard deviation of Y as follows:

$$\sqrt{\frac{24,149}{5} - (69.4)^2} = \sqrt{4,829.8 - 4,816.36} = \sqrt{13.44} = 3.67$$

$$r = \frac{\left(\dfrac{56,720}{5}\right) - 11,242.8}{(28.57 \times 3.67)} = \frac{11,344 - 11,242.8}{104.85} = \frac{101.2}{104.85} = 0.97$$

Another way to compute the Pearson r is by the mean deviation method (Runyon-Haber 1971). Using the same data, the Pearson r might be computed by the mean deviation method as shown in Table 7-10.

TABLE 7-9
Hypothetical Example of Pearson r Correlation Data

SUBJECT	WEIGHT (X)	X^2	HEIGHT (Y)	Y^2	$X \times Y$
A	170	28,900	72	5,184	12,240
B	140	19,600	66	4,356	9,240
C	120	14,400	64	4,096	7,680
D	180	32,400	72	5,184	12,960
E	200	40,000	73	5,329	14,600
Sums	810	135,300	347	24,149	56,720
Means	162		69.4		

TABLE 7-10
Hypothetical Example of Computation of Pearson r Using the Mean Deviation Method

SUBJECT	X	$X-\bar{X}$	$(X-\bar{X})^2$	Y	$Y-\bar{Y}$	$(Y-\bar{Y})^2$	$(X-\bar{X})(Y-\bar{Y})$
A	170	8	64	72	2.6	6.76	20.8
B	140	−22	484	66	−3.4	11.56	74.8
C	120	−42	1764	64	−5.4	29.16	226.8
D	180	18	324	72	2.6	6.76	46.8
E	200	38	1444	73	3.6	12.96	136.8
Sums	810	0	4080	347	0	67.20	506.0
Means	162			69.4			

$$r = \frac{506}{\sqrt{4,080 \times 67.2}} = \frac{506}{\sqrt{274,176}} = \frac{506}{523.62} = .97$$

Calculating the r both ways provides a check on our arithmetic. You may wish to use the method that is easiest for you. In our example, a correlation of .97 is a very high correlation, since it is close to 1. We can conclude that as height increases, weight increases. We might also express the findings in terms of: the taller one is, the more that person is likely to weigh.

INFERENTIAL STATISTICS

Inferential statistics are statistics we use to infer or draw a conclusion about something. We frequently want to know the probability of our sample representing the population. Probability is another word for chance. What are the chances that what we found is due to the research treatment and not just "luck"? If you flip a coin, the chance (or probability) of it turning up heads is 50 percent, or 0.50. How do we know that our treatment method is significantly less costly while being just as effective as a more traditional method? We might infer that one group of individuals is more likely to have certain attitudes than another group; for example, a group of nurses working in an oncology unit might have significantly different attitudes about caring for dying patients than nurses working in an obstetrics unit. With inferential statistics, we take what would otherwise be descriptive data and come to some conclusion.

An important concept of inferential statistics is *decision making.* Remember when we discussed hypotheses, we noted that the null hypothesis was a statement of "no difference." Although it seems strange to hypothesize no difference when we clearly want to show a difference to support our argument that our research is having an effect, the null hypothesis makes sense from a statistical point of view. In the next example (the chi square statistic), the null hypothesis is that there is no difference between the two groups on medication compliance. The attempt, therefore, is to disprove or reject the null hypothesis. If the obtained chi square had been less than 3.84, the null hypothesis could not have been rejected. The conclusion would have had to be that there was no difference between the groups, and the treatment was evidently not effective, at least on that variable.

There is, however, a possibility that even if the chi square value had been less than 3.84, the treatment might still have been effective. If it had been concluded that the treatment was not effective when it was, an error would have been committed that is known as a *Type II error.* A Type II error is defined as accepting the null hypothesis (of no difference) when the null hypothesis is false (i.e., when there really is a difference). *A Type I error* is possible in the example, since the null hypothesis was rejected and it was concluded that the treatment was effective. Maybe the treatment was not really effective; maybe other unknown variables were contaminating the data so that the null hypothesis was true. It is the possibility of committing these two types of errors that must be considered in statistical decision making. Table 7–11 illustrates the relationship of truth and errors in decision-making.

TABLE 7-11
Statistical Decision Making and Errors

| | | Truth | |
| | | Null Hypothesis | |
		True	False
Decision	Accept null hypothesis	Correct decision	Type II error
	Reject null hypothesis	Type I error	Correct decision

In nursing and other behaviorally oriented research concerned with people, a margin of error of .05 (the probability of making a Type I error and usually designated as *alpha* or α) is usually close enough (unless risk factors are involved). Compare this probability level with that of an engineer building a bridge. The engineer must not tolerate errors of measurement greater than 0.00001 or less (or you would not want to cross that bridge). Statistics provide us with tools for making decisions. Rarely (if ever) do we "prove" anything. We are only saying that, within an identified level of probability, we are willing to state that there was a difference.

If you are serious about the probability levels you establish for your research, you will avoid meaningless statements such as, "the data approached significance." Significance is an arbitrary level of probability established by the researcher (with regard to conventionally accepted practices by peers or as determined by theory).

In making decisions you need to know about *one-tailed* and *two-tailed* tests. If you are predicting direction—that is, if you believe that your treatment will reduce the number of hospital days as contrasted to simply being different from the number in the control group—you may use a one-tailed test. If you are not predicting direction, you must use a two-tailed test. The tails have to do with the distribution curve. A two-tailed test considers both ends of the curve (because neither end was specified). A one-tailed test only considers one end of the curve—the one that was predicted (hypothesized).

If you think about it, you will sense that it is more likely your test will be significant if you are only concerned with one tail rather than both. A two-tailed test is more conservative than a one-tailed test. It is important to use the one that is appropriate for your data.

Chi Square

As with descriptive and correlational statistics, the inferential statistic we choose depends on the type of data we collect. *Chi square* is an inferential statistic. You experienced the computation of chi square as part of the process in determining the contingency coefficient correlation earlier in this chapter. Chi square is appropriate for frequency data whenever you can count the number of items in a category. For example, suppose we wanted to compare a group of severely mentally disabled adults who are receiving intensive case coordination (experimental group) with a similar group of individuals who are receiving routine treatment (control group). The dependent variable is medication compliance. Set up a table as previously indicated for the contingency coefficient, as shown in Table 7-12.

TABLE 7-12
Hypothetical Data for Chi Square Statistic

TAKING MEDICATIONS AS PRESCRIBED	TYPE OF GROUP		
	EXPERIMENTAL	CONTROL	TOTALS
Yes	12 (8)	4 (8)	16
No	2 (6)	10 (6)	12
Totals	14	14	28

Recall that the way to obtain the expected values is to multiply the margin totals for each cell and divide by the total number of subjects.

$$14 \times 16 \div 28 = 8$$
$$14 \times 12 \div 28 = 6$$

The expected values are in parentheses in Table 7-12. To calculate chi square, subtract the expected value from the observed value, square the difference, and divide by the expected value as indicated below

$$(12 - 8)^2 = \quad (4) \times (4) = 16, 16/8 = 2$$
$$(4 - 8)^2 = (-4) \times (-4) = 16, 16/8 = 2$$
$$(2 - 6)^2 = (-4) \times (-4) = 16, 16/6 = 2.67$$
$$(10 - 6)^2 = \quad (4) \times (4) = 16, 16/6 = \underline{2.67}$$
$$\text{Chi square} = 9.34$$

Since the purpose of inferential statistics is to infer, in this case we want to know if the treatment of the experimental group results in those individuals being more likely to comply with medication prescriptions. To determine if there is a difference, we decide that if the probability of these data occurring by chance is less than 5 percent, we will assume the treatment is making the difference (since we have carefully controlled other variables and randomly assigned the subjects to the two groups).

We look up our obtained chi square value of 9.34 in a table using the degrees of freedom (*df*, a mathematical term related to the size of the sample but calculated differently in various formulas) as one minus the number of rows in our table multiplied by one minus the number of columns in our table. We have two rows and two columns. Two minus one is one; one times one is one. We enter the table in Appendix F at one *df* and note that the critical value for one degree of freedom at the 0.05 level of significance is 3.84. Since our chi square of 9.34 is greater than 3.84, we *reject* the null hypothesis. We conclude, therefore, that our intensive case coordination is resulting in a greater number of clients taking medications as prescribed; that is, the results are *statistically significant*.

Sign Test

A simple test that may be used with ordinal data is the *sign test*. Suppose in the case of the severely mentally disabled adults, the researcher matched each subject in the experimental group with a subject in the control group. We could use the sign test because, for each pair, we can determine which subject (experimental or control) was more compliant (took medication as prescribed more days in a given month). We might develop a table that looks like Table 7-13.

To determine the probability of these signs occurring by chance, count the signs. There are 4 minus signs. Look at the table in Appendix G. Since the number of fewer signs in our example is 4, $X = 4$. The number of matched pairs who showed differences was 14, so $N = 14$. The table in Appendix G shows a probability of 0.090 for $N = 14$ and $x \leq 4$. The value of 0.090 is not within the region of rejection of the null hypothesis; so using the sign test with these data, we cannot reject the null hypothesis, and we would conclude that our treatment is not making a difference. Since the outcomes, clinically, of the data used for the chi square and those used for the sign test are similar, why is one statistically significant and the other not? The results have to do with the power of the tests. Note that the sign test ignores a lot of data such as the size of the differences between each pair.

In general, the less stringent the test (fewer requirements for using it), the less powerful the test (the less likely you are to have significant results).

114

TABLE 7-13
Hypothetical Data for a Sign Test

SUBJECT PAIR	NUMBER OF DAYS TOOK MEDS EXPERIMENTAL	CONTROL	DIRECTION OF DIFFERENCE	SIGN
1	25	30	E < C	−
2	30	28	E > C	+
3	27	24	E > C	+
4	17	7	E > C	+
5	3	10	E < C	−
6	28	21	E > C	+
7	21	14	E > C	+
8	30	28	E > C	+
9	18	21	E < C	−
10	25	21	E > C	+
11	2	26	E < C	−
12	23	20	E > C	+
13	27	2	E > C	+
14	30	0	E > C	+

For that reason, it is an advantage to use the most stringent test for which your data can qualify. You should keep this in mind as you design your research project.

Mann-Whitney *U*

Even so, there are times when the assumptions required for the more powerful parametric inferential statistics cannot be met. In addition to the tests described above, the *Mann-Whitney U* is a nonparametric inferential statistical test that is appropriate for ordinal data. Siegel (1956) says of the Mann-Whitney *U* test that it is "one of the most powerful of the nonparametric tests, and it is a most useful alternate to the parametric *t* test when the researcher wishes to avoid the *t* test's assumptions, or when the measurement in the research is weaker than interval scaling" (p. 116).

Suppose we wanted to compare the subjects who took the attitudes-toward-elderly-individuals scale with a similar group in another geographic location where the ratio of individuals over 65 to the total population is higher than in our original sample used to illustrate the Spearman rho correlation. The research question might be: Is the attitude toward elderly individuals more positive in a population with a higher density of elderly individuals than in a population where the density of elderly individuals is lower? (Note that we have predicted direction and can, therefore, use a one-tailed test.)

The scores from group I (subjects from the lower density population) are 19, 5, 8, 14, 2, 6, 15, 3, 4, 10. The scores from group II (subjects from the higher density population) are: 24, 10, 13, 19, 7, 13, 22, 10, 11, 17. Note that these groups are *independent;* that is, there is no requirement for pairs or matching. To find U, rank the scores from both groups in order of increasing size while maintaining the identity of the group in the ranking, as illustrated in Table 7-14.

TABLE 7-14
Hypothetical Data to Illustrate Calculation of Mann-Whitney U

SCORE	GROUP	RANK
24	II	20
22	II	19
19	I	17.5
19	II	17.5
17	II	16
15	I	15
14	I	14
13	II	12.5
13	II	12.5
11	II	11
10	I	9
10	II	9
10	II	9
8	I	7
7	II	6
6	I	5
5	I	4
4	I	3
3	I	2
2	I	1

Count the number of scores made by subjects in group I that precede scores made by subjects in group II. Looking at Table 7-13, observe that the first score that appears from group I is 19 and it precedes eight scores from group II. The second group I score is 15, which precedes six group II scores. The third group I score is 14, which precedes six group II scores. The fourth score of 10 precedes three group II scores and the fifth score of 8 precedes one group II score. The remaining five group I scores do not precede any group II scores. To obtain the U score, add the number of group II scores preceded by group I scores: $8 + 6 + 6 + 3 + 1 = 24$.

Using the table in Appendix H, note that the critical value of U for a sample in which group I has ten subjects and group II has ten subjects is between 27 and 73. Our obtained U value in our hypothetical example is 24. Since our obtained value is outside the upper and lower limits of the critical region, we reject the null hypothesis and conclude that the attitudes toward elderly individuals were significantly more positive in the location where there was a higher concentration of individuals over 65 years old, when compared with a population of fewer elderly individuals per capita.

If you are curious about the upper limit of the U, you could calculate U'. To do so, follow the same procedure as used in calculating U by counting the number of times scores in group II precede scores in group I. You will notice that the first group II score is 24 and precedes ten group I scores. Likewise, the second group II score precedes ten group I scores; the third precedes nine scores; the fourth, nine scores; the fifth, seven scores; the sixth, seven scores; the seventh, seven scores; the eighth, six scores; the ninth, six scores; and the tenth, five scores.

$$U' = 10 + 10 + 9 + 9 + 7 + 7 + 7 + 6 + 6 + 5 = 76$$

Checking the table in Appendix H again, we notice that 76 is also outside the critical region. Our decision to reject the null hypothesis is confirmed.

t Test

The t test is a parametric test that is widely used. This test is sometimes referred to as *Student's t*. Since the t test is a parametric statistic, the assumptions that must be met include

1. Normal distribution—also referred to as a Gaussian distribution, a bell-shaped curve distribution, and is discussed earlier in this chapter under standard deviations.
2. Random sampling—discussed in Chapter 5.
3. Homogeneity of variance—indicating that the samples have the same variance. The F test is used for determining homogeneity of variance. The F test is considered a more advanced statistic and although widely used, it is not included in this text. In cases where the differences in variance is suspected, it would be important to determine whether there is a difference. This is because a "larger variance indicates more extreme scores at *both* ends of a distribution" (Runyon-Haber 1971, p. 200).

4. Independent samples—"the selection of any one case from the population for inclusion in the sample must not bias the chances of any other case for inclusion, and the score which is assigned to any case must not bias the score which is assigned to any other case" (Siegel 1956, p. 19).

5. Data measured on at least an interval scale—discussed throughout this chapter.

Although these assumptions seem rather stringent, Siegel (1956) indicates "these conditions are ordinarily not tested in the course of the performance of a statistical analysis. Rather, they are presumptions which are accepted, and their truth or falsity determines the meaningfulness of the probability statement arrived at by the parametric test" (p. 19–20).

For an example of the t test, go back to the hypothetical study of infants whose mothers were given a food supplement during the third trimester of pregnancy. To determine (infer) if the supplement made a difference, it would be necessary to compare this experimental group to a control group—one who got a regular diet. Table 7-15 shows the lengths in inches of the infants in the experimental (X) and control (Y) groups.

TABLE 7-15
Hypothetical Data for Illustration of the t Test

	EXPERIMENTAL GROUP		CONTROL GROUP	
	X	X^2	Y	Y^2
	18	324	18	324
	19	361	18	324
	19	361	19	361
	19	361	18	324
	19	361	20	400
	20	400	18	324
	20	400	19	361
	21	441	17	289
	22	484	21	441
	23	529	20	400
Sums	200	4,022	188	3,548
Means	20		18.8	

First calculate the sum of squares for each group. Take the sum of the squared data (4,022 for the experimental group) and subtract the sum of the Xs squared divided by the number of subjects.

$$4{,}022 - \frac{(200)^2}{10}$$

$$4{,}022 - (40{,}000/10) = 22$$

Repeat the procedure to obtain the sum of squares for the control group

$$3{,}548 - \frac{(188)^2}{10}$$

$$3{,}548 - (35{,}344/10) = 13.6$$

Using the sum of squares just calculated, obtain the pooled estimate of the standard error of the difference between the means. This figure is the square root of the sum of the sums of squares divided by the number of subjects (10) in each group multiplied by the number of subjects minus 1 (9, in the example).

$$\sqrt{\frac{(22 + 13.6)}{90}} = \sqrt{\frac{35.6}{90}} = .63$$

(This procedure is only appropriate when the number of subjects is the same in both groups.)

The t is obtained by subtracting the mean of the control group (18.8) from the mean of the experimental group (20) and dividing by the pooled estimate of the standard error of difference between means.

$$(20 - 18.8) / .63 = (1.2 / .63) = 1.9$$

The total degrees of freedom for the two-sample case is the sum of the number of subjects in both samples minus 2.

$$df = 10 + 10 - 2 = 18$$

Enter the table in Appendix I for 18 degrees of freedom at the 0.05 level of significance for a one-tailed test. You should find that the critical value is 1.734. Since our obtained value of 1.9 is greater than 1.734, we can reject the null hypothesis and consider recommending the food supplement (assuming there are no undesirable side effects such as indigestion or excessive weight gain for the mother, that the cost is not prohibitive, and that we want longer babies).

Statistical Significance of Correlation

The *statistical significance of correlations* can also be determined. The correlations, as we calculated them, only showed us the strength of the relationship but did not show levels of significance. So we were not able to determine if the relationship occurred as a result of chance or if the relationship was significant.

For the contingency coefficient correlation, it is possible to determine whether the observed value differs significantly from chance by deciding if the chi square for the data is significant (Siegel 1956). In our example of contingency coefficient earlier in this chapter, chi square was 15.05. The degrees of freedom are determined (as indicated earlier in this chapter) by multiplying the number of columns minus one times the number of rows minus one.

$$(6-1) \ (4-1) = 15 \text{ degrees of freedom}$$

The table in Appendix F indicates that the critical value of chi square for 15 degrees of freedom is 25. Since our obtained chi square in *less than* the critical value, our contingency coefficient is not statistically significant.

The Spearman *rho* correlation example earlier in this chapter had a value of −.66 for ten pairs (ten subjects measured on two variables). The table in Appendix J indicates a critical value of .564 at the .05 level of probability. Since our obtained *rho* is greater than .564, we reject the null hypothesis and say that SES is inversely related to attitudes toward elderly individuals. (Note that the absolute value of the *rho* is used in comparing it with the critical value in the table. The fact that the calculated *rho* is negative does not make it less than the critical value.)

For our calculated Pearson product moment correlation, we could guess that our *r* is significant because .97 is close to a perfect correlation. A look at the table in Appendix K confirms our impressions. The critical value of *r* for three degrees of freedom is .8783 at the .05 level of significance. The degrees of freedom for correlation coefficients are equal to the number of subjects minus 2 (Polit and Hungler 1978). Our observed value of .97 is greater than the critical value. We can reject the null hypothesis and state that height and weight are significantly correlated. Not to be facetious, but even with a correlation as high as this, it does *not* mean that if I gain weight I will grow taller. Interpretations of statistics, even when significant, must be done cautiously.

SUMMARY

Statistics provides tools for organizing and analyzing data. The statistical tests employed are no more useful than the quality of the data being tested. The quality of the data is no better than the quality of the research design. Much emphasis is placed on statistics in evaluating research. Some of the emphasis is because individuals do not appreciate the limitations of statistics; others emphasize statistics because they appreciate the limitations.

How to present your findings and what interpretations you can make of them are the topics for discussion in the next chapter. After you have finished the process, you have some responsibility for making recommendations for nursing practice and for further research. Recommendations will also be a part of Chapter 8.

Suggestions for Further Study

1. Follow up on the study you chose for number one of "Suggestions for Further Study" from Chapter 4 by identifying the type of statistics used in the article. Specifically, were they descriptive, inferential, or correlational statistics? What level of probability was used for determining significance for inferential statistics? Did the data represent nominal, ordinal, interval, or ratio scales? Were the tests used appropriate for the level of the data? Was a null hypothesis stated? If so, was it rejected? Why, or why not?

2. For the project you are working on, identify the level of data you are collecting. Is your study descriptive, correlational, or experimental? Which statistical test will you use? Give rationale for your decision.

3. When you have your data, analyze it appropriately and discuss it with peers and faculty.

4. Go to the nearest computer center with your data and ask someone to show you how to input your data and obtain the analyzed results. You will need to be able to summarize your study for the statistician or computer person so that you get appropriate instructions to obtain meaningful results. *You* know your study; they merely know statistics and computers.

Suggestions for Additional Reading

Brogan, D. "Choosing an Appropriate Statistical Test of Significance for a Nursing Research Hypothesis or Question," *Western Journal of Nursing Research,* 1981, *3*(4), pp. 337–369.

Edwards, A. L. *Statistical Analysis* (revised ed.). New York: Holt, Rinehart and Winston, 1958.

Hays, W. L. *Statistics.* New York: Holt, Rinehart and Winston, 1963.

Huff, D. *How to Lie with Statistics.* New York: W. W. Norton & Company, Inc., 1954.

Knapp, R. G. *Basic Statistics for Nurses.* New York: John Wiley & Sons, 1978.

Polit, D. F., and Hungler, B. P. *Nursing Research: Principles and Methods* (2nd edition). Philadelphia: J. B. Lippincott Company, 1983.

Runyon, R. P., and Haber, A. *Fundamentals of Behavioral Statistics* (2nd edition). Reading, MA: Addison-Wesley Publishing Company, 1971.

Siegel, S. *Nonparametric Statistics: For the Behavioral Sciences.* New York: McGraw-Hill Book Company, 1956.

Waltz, C. F., and Bausell, R. B. *Nursing Research: Design, Statistics and Computer Analysis.* Philadelphia: F. A. Davis Company, 1981.

Chapter 8

What sense are you going to make of it?

FINDINGS, INTERPRETATIONS, AND RECOMMENDATIONS

Chapter Objectives

Upon successful completion of this chapter the student will be able to

- Distinguish between findings and interpretations
- Present findings in a logical order
- Define and identify serendipitous findings
- Make interpretations of findings that are significant in the expected direction, significant in the opposite direction, and inconclusive
- Differentiate between summary and conclusions
- Make recommendations based on the findings of a study

INTRODUCTION

You have your data, you have organized it and analyzed it. What does it all mean? Another heading appropriate for this section would be "fact, meanings, and suggested actions," as discussed by Wandelt (1970). You present the data (facts), make some interpretations of these facts according to your purpose and research questions (meanings), and make recommendations based on the conclusions you draw from all that has preceded (suggested actions).

There should be no surprises here. A research endeavor is logical and consistent. You would not build an office building and put a church steeple on it. Likewise, you do not do a study about postoperative nursing care and make interpretations about surgical procedures. That does not mean that the view from the top of the office building might not be different from what was expected or that the postoperative study does not serendipitously reveal something about surgical procedures.

You will probably find this chapter dull if you have not actually followed the preceding chapters while doing an investigation, *at least* hypothetically. Abbott (1981) suggested that the most creative and demanding part of conducting research is in reporting the findings, conclusions, and recommendations. Abbott referred to the findings as "buried treasure" (p. 129). So if you are not excited about findings and what they mean, go find some buried treasure to relate to, or read this quotation from Meyer and Heidgerken (1962) and be inspired (after overcoming any reaction to the generic use of the male pronouns).

> The researcher occupies a unique position in the society of men. He stands on the bridge of time and scans the passing world. His work may have been started in the remote past and may be shared in the future by people as yet unborn. And he is wary of the present, which underwrites his activities, prods him for solutions, is offered as his guinea pig, and is critical of his indecisive character but will quickly absorb the fruits of his labors. (p. 408)

PRESENTATION OF FINDINGS

The presentation of findings involves *what* to present and the *order* of presentation. As you write a research report, you will want to provide an introduction to this section to remind your readers of the purpose of the study so that the findings are more meaningful. The contents to be included in the presentation of findings are a *description of the subjects*, the *data* as gathered to address the research questions (or hypotheses), and any *serendipitous* (*unexpected*) information you happened to come across. The presentation is factual, meaning that value judgments, apologies, or triumphs are not expressed. All of the data you collected should be reported. (If it does not relate to your study, you should not have gathered it. The temptation to "just see" what might be there should be avoided.)

Description of Sample

In describing the subjects who comprised your sample, be sure to include the obvious—how many there were. If you had more than one group, describe each group. Include demographic characteristics such as age, sex, race, income, education, ethnic background, location of residence (rural or urban), and/or other characteristics you gathered about the subjects. Remember to refer to the subjects as "subjects" and not patients, students, children, or any other label. Once you have admitted individuals to your study, they become "subjects." Tables are useful for presenting *descriptive data*. (The information about the subjects is referred to as descriptive data.) The following excerpt from a master's thesis illustrates several points.

EXCERPT 8-1

THE RELATIONSHIP BETWEEN SCHOOL-AGE EPILEPTIC CHILDREN'S KNOWLEDGE OF THEIR DISEASE AND THEIR SELF-CONCEPT

THE SAMPLE

The sample for this study consisted of 14 children who were receiving outpatient health care at a state funded seizure clinic located in a southeastern metropolitan area. Selected demographic characteristics of the subjects are presented in Table 1.

As shown in Table 1, the subjects consisted of five females and nine males. The mean age was 9.99 years with a range of 5 years. Five of the children were black, while nine were white. All of the subjects had been seen regularly at the seizure clinic and, at the time of the study, were accompanied by a parent, grandparent, aunt, or legal guardian. All of the subjects who consented to participate in the study did so without any withdrawals. The mean age at the time of diagnosis was 4.58 years with a range from 1 to 9.5 years in age. As shown in Table 1, there was no pattern to the ages at the time of diagnosis. However, 7 subjects were above the mean age when diagnosed, and 7 were below the mean. Information related to seizure type, anticonvulsant medication, and seizure frequency are found in Table 2.

TABLE 1
Demographic Data

SUBJECT	AGE[a]	SEX[b]	RACE[c]	AGE AT TIME OF DIAGNOSIS
3	7.5	F	W	5.6
1	7.75	M	W	5.5
7	7.75	F	B	1.0
2	8.08	F	W	6.08
6	8.08	M	W	4.0
12	9.75	M	W	2.5
13	10.0	M	W	3.0
11	10.08	M	W	3.0
9	10.4	F	W	1.5
5	11.5	M	B	9.5
14	11.8	M	W	6.0
4	12.3	F	B	8.4
8	12.3	M	B	6.0
10	12.5	M	B	2.0
Means	9.99			4.58

[a] Age is in years   [b] M = male; F = female   [c] W = White; B = Black

TABLE 2
Type of Seizure, Anticonvulsant Medication, and Time since Last Seizure

SUBJECT	SUBJECT TYPE[a]	MEDICATION[b]	LAST SEIZURE[c]
13	T. C.	Dil	1
3	T. C.	P	3
8	T. C.	Dil	3
5	T. C.	P	6
2	T. C.	P	6
1	T. C.	P	24
14	T. C.	P	24
9	T. C.	P, Dil	36
4	P. M.	P, Dil	1
10	P. M.	Dil, Teg	1
12	P. M.	P, Dil, Teg	3
6	T. C./P. M.	P, Dil, Teg	1
11	T. C./P. M.	P, Dil	1
7	T. C./Petit Mal	P, Dil, Z	1
		mean =	7.93

[a] T. C. = Tonic-clonic; P. M. = psychomotor
[b] P = Phenobarbital; Dil = Dilantin; Z = Zarontin; Teg = Tegretol
[c] Time is measured in months

The seizure type varied among the subjects, but as shown in Table 2, 11 out of the 14 subjects had tonic-clonic seizures, 5 out of 14 subjects had psychomotor, 1 out of 14 had petit mal, and 3 out of 14 had a combination of two types. All of the subjects were currently on one or more of the anticonvulsant medications. Type of anticonvulsants taken by the subjects were Phenobarbital, Dilantin, Zarontin, and Tegretol. The amount of time lapsed since the subjects' last seizures, which was measured in monthly increments, showed a mean of 7.93 months with a range from 1 to 36 months. Eleven subjects, however, were considerably below the mean.

According to the data shown in Table 2, the children with tonic-clonic seizures required a less complex medication regimen for control and also demonstrated a better record of seizure control than the children who had another type of seizure or a combination of types of seizures. Six out of 8 of the children with tonic-clonic seizures had been seizure free 6 months or more and 3 out of 8 of the children with tonic-clonic seizures had been seizure free 24 to 36 months. None of the subjects with psychomotor seizures or combinations of seizure types had been seizure free longer than 3 months.

There are several points to be made from Excerpt 8-1.

1. The number of subjects is stated in the first sentence.
2. Although the subjects are called children in the first sentence, the term is used there as a description of the sample. Later in the excerpt (last paragraph) the author, incorrectly, referred to the subjects as "children."
3. The setting for the study is indicated in the description of the clinic where the subjects were receiving care.
4. The identity of the clinic is kept anonymous to preserve the rights of the subjects as well as the clinic.
5. The demographic characteristics and other data relevant to the study are presented clearly in tables.
6. Each table is introduced, presented, and followed with a discussion of the data contained in the table.
7. The tables are numbered with Arabic numerals consecutively, and each table has a title that communicates the contents of the table.

(This form may vary depending on the writing style being used, but the form for tables should be consistent throughout a manuscript.)

8. Superscripts are used to indicate the definition of the terms of the legend.

9. Columns (vertical—columns support) are appropriately labeled.

10. Horizontal rules are used effectively to separate headings from data and data from summary and legend.

11. The author chose to arrange the data in ascending order according to age. This order causes the subjects' assigned numbers to be out of order but makes more sense.

12. Tables are not crowded with confusing information. For example, the author has two tables instead of trying to squeeze the two into one. Although both tables contain descriptive information about the subjects, the type of information is sufficiently different to mandate the use of two separate tables.

13. Information in the tables is appropriately summarized when possible in the tables. For example, the means of the ages and times since the last seizure are presented.

14. Ages and time are ratio data and, therefore, means are appropriate measures of central tendency.

15. In the discussion that follows each table, the author presents the information in a different way than was presented in the tables. It is not simply a repetition but a different look at the same data; the relationship of types of seizures and time since last seizure, for example, instead of just the raw data, as in the tables. The text has to stand alone and the table has to stand alone—each comprehensible in itself.

16. No opinions or value judgments are made in the discussion. There are implications to be sure, but they are left to the reader or to the researcher to comment on in a later section. Everything presented here is fact.

17. Numbers 10 and above are written as Arabic numerals while those below 10 and those at the beginning of a sentence are written as words. Ages are written as numbers even when they are below 10. The beginning of a sentence is still another exception; never begin a sentence with a number. It is suggested in the *Publication Manual of the American Psychological Association* (1983) that whenever possible, sentences should be rewritten so that they do not begin with numbers.

Presentation and Analysis of Data

The order of the presentation is important. Begin with your first hypothesis. Present the data gathered to test that hypothesis. Go on to the next hypothesis. State each hypothesis before you present the data. Use tables or figures whenever they would help to clarify or illustrate the data. Identify each tool used for gathering the data and the statistical tests used for analyzing the data. The mathematical calculations are not shown, but advisors of beginning researchers frequently want enough details to make it possible to check the work. Raw data may be included in an appendix of a report. Always report the level of probability chosen for significance. Although researchers will disagree, it is interesting to report the actual probability obtained if you are using a computer or other means of calculating exact probabilities (in contrast to using tables to determine only whether or not an obtained value falls within the acceptable range of confidence). For the purpose of illustration, another excerpt from the same thesis as Excerpt 8-1 will be used.

EXCERPT 8-2

THE RELATIONSHIP BETWEEN SCHOOL AGE EPILEPTIC CHILDREN'S KNOWLEDGE OF THEIR DISEASE AND THEIR SELF-CONCEPT

PRESENTATION OF DATA

A descriptive, correlational design was used in this study. This design was used in order to examine the potential relationships between school age epileptic children's knowledge of their disease and their self-concept. The interview schedule was administered in order to attempt to measure the subject's knowledge of epilepsy. The possible scores on the knowledge tool ranged from 1 to 27 with a higher score indicating more knowledge of the disease. Scores from the interview schedule and the Piers-Harris Self-concept Scale can be found in Table 3.

As shown in Table 3, the mean knowledge score was 18.14 with a range of 11 points from 13 to 24 points. Eight subjects scored below the mean, while 6 scored above the mean.

Upon scoring the interview schedule, the researcher found that some of the questions actually measured affective response rather than knowledge. The questions indicating affective responses were then scored separately with a higher score reflecting greater emotional responses. The maximum

TABLE 3
Interview Schedule and Piers-Harris Self-concept Scale Scores

SUBJECT	INTERVIEW SCHEDULE KNOWLEDGE SCORES	INTERVIEW SCHEDULE EMOTIONAL SCORES	PIERS-HARRIS SELF-CONCEPT SCALE SCORES[a]
3	13	3	57
7	13	2	71
13	13	2	74
6	14	8	45
1	16	2	53
4	17	6	42
14	17	1	67
9	18	9	43
11	21	2	34
12	21	4	56
10	21	7	63
5	22	2	40
2	24	5	32
8	24	9	52
Means	18.14	4.43	52.07
Max[b]	27	10	80

[a] Standardized average is 46 to 60
[b] Max = maximum score possible

possible score for affective responses was 10. The mean score was 4.43 with a range of 8 points from 1 to 9. Five subjects scored about the mean for emotional responses.

The second tool used in the study was the Piers-Harris Children's Self-concept Scale to test the first hypothesis. That instrument is scored according to the number of correct responses. Thus, the higher the raw score, the higher the self-concept. Average scores are considered to be those between 46 to 60 (Piers-Harris, 1969). The mean score for subjects in this study was 52.07 with a range of 42 points from 32 to 74. In the sample, 6 out of 14 scored below the reported average of 46 to 60 and 4 out of 14 scored above the reported average. However, the mean score for these subjects was within the reported average of 46 to 60.

The researcher continued the presentation of the data with further description of the attributes measured by the Piers-Harris Self-concept Scale. She described the administration and data gathered from a third tool. For the purpose of illustration look back at the excerpt presented and consider the following points.

1. The researcher chose to separate the presentation and the analysis of the data. By separating the two parts, the author was able to make the presentation of detailed data more clear than might have been possible otherwise. Whether or not such detail is necessary or desirable is a value judgment and depends on the purpose and guidelines of the report.

2. The type of design used is indicated. It is recognized that the type of design was identified under methodology; the repetition here serves as a reminder as the researcher pulls the study together. Think of a drawstring gathering a parcel; you want to make sure that all areas are included as you prepare the package for delivery.

3. In the second sentence, the term "potential" is inappropriate because a descriptive study is conducted to describe what is, not what is potential.

4. The type of instrument used is identified, and the fact that the researcher collected all of the data is important for consistency.

5. Finding that the interview measured affective responses rather than knowledge raises two questions: (a) Why was such an evaluation not left until the discussion section? (b) Why was pilot study not done prior to the study so that such a problem could have been avoided? The basis for the reported finding is not clear.

6. The author chose to organize Table 3 with the Interview Schedule Knowledge Scores in ascending order and the other data falling into place around that item.

7. When the author referred to "the first hypothesis," it would have been helpful if she had repeated the hypothesis. The reader does not know what the hypotheses were. It is not unusual, by the way, to read the data presentation section before reading the first part of a study. If there are specific facts you want to know, you go to the section most likely to have those facts. You need not start at the beginning of the report.

8. To write that the "Piers-Harris Self-concept Scale is a 15–20 minute self-report instrument" sounds as though the instrument does the reporting on itself in that length of time. What is meant is that the subjects usually require 15–20 minutes to complete the Piers-Harris Self-concept Scale.

9. At this point, I am tired of writing "Piers-Harris Self-concept Scale" and an abbreviation would be acceptable (even desirable). To abbreviate, simply write the abbreviation in parentheses after the full name has been written out once. From that point, the abbreviation alone will suffice; for example, Piers-Harris Self-concept Scale (PH-SCS).

10. "Between 46 to 60" should be expressed "between 46 *and* 60" or "from 46 to 60."

Note in Excerpt 8-2 that the data are only presented. You are told nothing about the statistical significance of the findings. Separating presentation from analysis is an option and the decision depends on the form and extent of the data, the complexity of the study, and the preference and writing style of the researcher. It is easier to successfully combine sections in simpler studies than in more complex ones.

The author chose to separate the presentation of the data and the analysis. An excerpt from the data analysis section will be helpful in illustrating how the analysis might be presented.

EXCERPT 8-3

THE RELATIONSHIP BETWEEN SCHOOL AGE EPILEPTIC CHILDREN'S KNOWLEDGE OF THEIR DISEASE AND THEIR SELF-CONCEPT

ANALYSIS OF DATA

The data in this study were obtained from three sources: the results of the interview schedule on knowledge of epilepsy; the scores from the Piers-Harris Self-concept Scale; and, the scores from the HFDs [*Human Figure Drawings*]. The results of the interview schedule and the results from the self-concept scale were then used to test the first hypothesis. The researcher's first hypothesis proposed that a relationship does exist between school age epileptic children's knowledge of their disease and their self-concept as measured by the Piers-Harris Self-concept Scale. These data were analyzed using the Pearson r correlation coefficient. The results showed a negative correlation ($-.55$) which was significant ($p < .05$). This correlation indicates an inverse relation between the subjects' knowledge of epilepsy and their self-concepts; the researcher's hypothesis was supported and the null hypothesis was rejected.

Data from Koppitz Evaluation of Children's Human Figure Drawings were used to test the second hypothesis. The second null hypothesis said that there was no relationship between school age epileptic children's knowledge of their disease and their self-concept as measured by Koppitz Evaluation of Children's HFDs. The researcher's hypothesis said that a relationship did exist. Neither the results from analysis of the knowledge scores and the Developmental Items scores (.42) nor the knowledge scores and the Emotional Indicators (−.48) were significant ($p > .05$). The data were further analyzed according to age, sex, and race. The relationship between age and knowledge (.47) for the sample as a whole was not found to be significant ($p > .05$). When separated by sex, it was found that the boys' ages and their knowledge of epilepsy showed a significant ($p < .05$) positive correlation (.60). When separated by race, the black children demonstrated a significant ($p < .05$) positive (.74) correlation when age was compared with knowledge level. The white children, on the other hand, showed a very low, positive (.16) correlation which was not significant when compared on the same two variables.

The subjects were then divided into two groups according to age. The first group included subjects between 7.5 and 10.0 years of age, while the second group included subjects between 10.08 and 12.5 years of age.

When the relationship between knowledge and self-concept was explored for the two separate age groups, the younger subjects showed a significant ($p < .05$) negative correlation (−.70). The older subjects did not show a statistically significant relationship. Neither age group showed a significant relationship, however, between knowledge and their scores on the HFDs.

[Other analyses were similarly presented.]

In summary, statistically significant findings were demonstrated for the researcher's first hypothesis which proposed that a relationship exists between school age epileptic children's knowledge of their disease and their self-concept as measured by the Piers-Harris Self-concept Scale. Thus, the researcher's first hypothesis was supported by the Pearson *r* coefficient.

On the other hand, the data did not support the researcher's second hypothesis. The researcher's second hypothesis stated that a statistically significant relationship exists between school age epileptic children's knowledge of their disease and their self-concept as measured by Koppitz Evaluation of children's HFDs. Thus the second null hypothesis was not rejected. Some significant relationships were also demonstrated in the secondary data.

Based on Excerpt 8-3, the following points about data analysis are made.

1. It is inconsistent to fail to capitalize one tool (that is, refer to it informally), present another by full name with first letters capitalized, and abbreviate the third one. The title in brackets for HFDs is this author's so that you will know what is meant.

2. The hypotheses being tested are stated here.

3. The author does not identify the level of the data (whether nominal, ordinal, interval, or ratio). Therefore, it is not clear that the Pearson r correlation coefficient was the appropriate statistic.

4. The degrees of freedom used for determining whether the obtained r was significant should have been specified. The reader can figure it out by going back to the previous section and determining how many subjects were in the study, but this exercise should not be necessary.

5. Note that the first hypothesis was "two-tailed," since the author did not specify the expected direction of the relationship, that is, whether the relationship was expected to be positive or negative.

6. The author could have postponed the interpretation of the inverse relationship of knowledge and self-concept, but for many beginning readers of research this sentence helps to clarify the results of this analysis.

7. Do we assume that "Developmental Items" refers to the Koppitz Evaluation of HFDs? We are, no doubt, at a disadvantage because we do not have the description of this scale. Even with that consideration, it is important not to change terms. The beginning research reporter typically believes it is not literarily pleasing to use the same term repeatedly. In research, however, it is necessary to use the same term for consistency and clarity or to define as such any words used as synonyms.

8. A better way of reporting the data would be "Black subjects demonstrated a significant positive correlation of age and knowledge ($r = .74$, $df = 5$, $p < .05$)." Actually, there is an error somewhere since p is greater than .05 for this r and df. If the author had reported the df she was using and the rationale, we might be more comfortable with the analysis of the data.

9. The *subjects* were not divided into two groups according to age, as the author reports; the *data* (or scores) were divided according to the subjects' ages. Learning to be concrete and literal is necessary for research reporting.

10. Some of the correlation coefficient values that were not significant were not reported. This practice is acceptable, but consistency is de-

sirable. Either report only significant r values (those where $p < .05$) or report *all* r values. To report some that are not significant and not report others that are also not significant does not make sense.

11. The summary is succinct with both hypotheses addressed.

12. You should have some questions about the analysis of the data because you do not have sufficient information to understand why the author used two measures of self-concept; whether she wanted to determine which was the "better" measure; and, if so, whether "better" means diagnostic (measuring how the child feels about himself or herself now) or predictive (how the child is likely to cope with the disease over a period of time, as through adolescence).

13. The author has overused possessive forms of words. This problem is particularly evident in the summary where she has "researcher's" (times four), "children's" (times three), and "their" (times four). Readability could be enhanced by reordering the sentences so that most (some would say all) of the possessive forms of words could be eliminated.

Serendipitous Findings

Any noteworthy data that emerge as a result of your investigation, but were not directly addressed in your hypotheses or research questions, are serendipitous or unexpected findings. Some strict researchers and statisticians will advise you to omit anything that you did not explicitly search for. There are some good reasons for the strict approach: if you did not design your study to specifically investigate a certain phenomenon, you did not have appropriate conditions for collecting those data. A more lenient approach is appropriate for several reasons: data collected in nursing studies are usually obtained in a complex setting where the investigator has ample opportunity to make other observations during the process of data collecting; in analyzing complex data, other relationships occur to the researcher who has the obligation to check out those relationships in the data at hand; often the data obtained are not statistically significant, but observation and reporting of serendipitous findings will often be useful in clarifying the limitations of the design; and, most important, it is frequently through the serendipitous findings that ideas for further research emerge. After all, such important phenomena as penicillin and X-rays were serendipitous findings.

An example of differences of opinion about reporting data occurred in a study of surviving spouses of individuals who had died of cancer. The researcher interviewed the spouses and found many more interesting facts than those relating to the research questions. The statistician consultant advised the researcher to quantify the data relating to the questions only. The researcher believed that such a move would reduce the potential value of the study by eliminating much valuable information. It is important for further research, for example, to know that surviving spouses welcomed the opportunity to talk with a nurse about the experiences surrounding the deaths of their spouses. It is also useful to know that the interviews took more than twice as long as expected because the subjects wanted to talk; to have left them without that opportunity seemed inappropriate and, indeed, unethical. The researcher chose to include the serendipitous findings in that study, and subsequent nurse researchers have been grateful.

Instead of having a separate section for serendipitous findings, the author of the previously reported excerpts chose to combine all of her findings under the two headings, Presentation of Data and Analysis of Data. The advantage of separating serendipitous findings from the data explicitly sought is that you can highlight your hypotheses and research questions more clearly if the data are separated. Except for clarity, whether to combine or separate makes no big difference.

INTERPRETATION OF FINDINGS

The interpretation of the findings (also known as the *discussion*) is presented in the order of the hypotheses or research questions. Having presented the reasons for your study, the conceptual framework within which you are working, the method by which you obtained the data, the data, and the analysis of those data, you are now ready to make some interpretations about what you found. While this section is the most creative because it is less structured, it must still be based on previous information or the speculations must be logical. Your data are likely to fall into one of the following categories: statistically significant as hypothesized; statistically significant in the opposite direction of the research hypothesis; not statistically significant. As Polit and Hungler (1978) wrote: "There is no such thing as a study whose results 'came out the wrong way,' if the 'wrong way' is the truth" (p. 602).

When the Findings are Statistically Significant in the Predicted Direction

This event is the happy outcome. There are many assumptions implied in the presentation of findings that are statistically significant. First, there is the assumption that your hypothesis was logically formulated and empirically testable. It is also assumed that your design was appropriate for your hypothesis, that you controlled the variables appropriately, you gathered the data and analyzed them accurately using the appropriate statistics, and that your level of significance was appropriate (.05, or with some logical explanation for anything different). Having met each of these assumptions, you are in the position of being able to reject the null hypothesis; that is, you have demonstrated that there is a difference and that difference cannot be attributed solely to chance. Are you sure that it was the experimental manipulation of the variables that contributed to the difference? If so, how much of that difference did the manipulation contribute? These questions can be addressed in light of the literature, the conceptual framework, and the design.

Use a straightforward approach in interpreting your significant findings. Avoid overstatement; do not go beyond what was actually tested. Do not minimize your findings either. How do your findings compare with the literature? Be specific. You are in agreement with which points in the literature? There is probably some literature that is contrary to your findings. Report those opposing views also. Why do you think your findings were different from those previously reported? What about your conceptual framework? How do your findings support or raise questions about your conceptual framework? It is assumed that if your findings are statistically significant, you are in agreement with most of the literature you reviewed and with the conceptual framework you chose. So the burden is to discuss how your study lends support to the conceptual framework.

Although the discussion has been primarily related to experimental research, investigators using nonexperimental designs have similar responsibility to discuss significant findings in light of the theory and literature. If there is a difference in two populations you observed, you must have suspected a difference or you would not have done the study. What does the difference mean? Did the literature reviewed contain evidences that differences would exist? Did the conceptual framework provide clues that these differences might exist? Remember to be specific. To report that the findings support the literature is not sufficient—specify precisely what facts reported in the literature are supported by your findings.

When the Findings Are Statistically Significant in the Opposite Direction of That Hypothesized

While findings that are the opposite of the predictions may be devastating, depending on the nature of your study, these may be the most interesting findings of all. For some reason, things are not happening in the way you expected. What are those reasons? You cannot ignore these data—something has to be done with them. Are nurses practicing some procedure that is actually detrimental to health instead of improving clients' conditions significantly? How are you going to account for your unexpected (but *not* serendipitous) findings? Examine your literature—how is your study different from the ones previously reported? Different age groups? Different geographical locations which might have a different climate and exposure to elements? Different agency policies? Reexamine the study design and procedure to detect possible biases or alternative explanations for the results. Scrutinize each possibility carefully.

Examine the conceptual framework. Was it appropriate for your study? Why or why not? If so, what was it that you misinterpreted that led you to make the wrong prediction? If not, what would be a better framework? "Better" means more accurately predictive. Find a framework that is consistent with your findings and trace logically how it provides a better foundation for your research problem.

When the Findings Are Inconclusive

What does it mean when the findings are not significant? First, decide if your sample was adequate. If no fault can be found with the sample, face the fact that there might not be a difference. If findings in the opposite direction are the most interesting, inconclusive findings are the most frustrating. Abbott (1981) suggests that "instead of saying, the investigator failed to demonstrate a relationship between X and Y, a better statement would be, it was demonstrated that the hypothesized relationship does not exist between X and Y" (p. 131). A preferable viewpoint is Meyer and Heidgerken's (1962) admonition that "the researcher should not discard the hypothesis hastily. . . . The possibility may exist, for example, that unnoticed but relevant factors were present to influence the results systematically rather than randomly" (p. 412). Similarly, Kerlinger (1964) pointed out that

> any weak link in the research chain can cause negative results. . . . If, for example, a weak nonparametric test is used when a strong parametric one is needed, an actual relation can go undetected. . . . If we can be fairly sure that the methodology, the measurement, and analysis are adequate, then negative results can be definite contributions to scientific advance, since then and only then can we have some confidence that our hypotheses are not correct. (pp. 620–621)

If you are convinced and present a convincing argument that your study meets the criteria as suggested by Kerlinger (1964), then report your nonsignificant findings as demonstrating no relationship. If, however, you have some reasonable doubt about *any* link in the research chain, report that your findings failed to demonstrate a relationship.

A recent example of a study reported in which this dilemma existed is the article by Lim-Levy (1982). This study was designed to "determine the effect of oxygen inhalation by nasal cannula on oral temperatures" (p. 150). The analysis of the data showed no statistically significant change in temperatures regardless of oxygen treatment. Lim-Levy reported "This study did not show a significant effect of oxygen inhalation on oral temperature" (p. 152).

For further illustration, since the author of the previous three excerpts obtained both significant and nonsignificant results, attention will be given to her discussion.

EXCERPT 8-4

THE RELATIONSHIP BETWEEN SCHOOL AGE EPILEPTIC CHILDREN'S KNOWLEDGE OF THEIR DISEASE AND THEIR SELF-CONCEPT

DISCUSSION

The presentation and analysis of the data from the research study demonstrate the relationship between school age epileptic children's knowledge of their disease and their self-concept as measured by two distinct tools. The following elaboration on the results, the strengths and weaknesses of the tools, and the statistical manipulation of the findings will interpret the significance of the data in relation to this study. In addition, certain supplementary findings will be discussed.

A noteworthy characteristic of the relationship between the epileptic children's knowledge of their disease and their self-concept is that a negative correlation was proven. Interpreting this finding, one notes that as the level of knowledge increased, the subjects' self-concept decreased. The researcher believes that there are several possible explanations for this inverse relationship: (1) the education that these childdren have received about their disease may have emphasized the abnormality and thus left the children with a negative connotation of their disease process; (2) greater understanding of their disease and the necessary treatment, enhances these children's perceptions of loss of control over their bodies; and, (3) the increased level of knowledge regarding epilepsy, contributes to these children's realization of their dissimilarity from their peers.

The researcher believes that the type of education given to epileptic children is important. These children should be helped to understand their roles in control of their seizures by compliance with their medication regimen, by recognizing an acceptable level of activity, and by recognizing the stimulus for their seizures. Epileptic children need to be encouraged to live as nearly a normal life as is realistically possible. Children with any illness need to have their normality rather than their disease emphasized.

The data also support the need for intervention in dealing with emotional problems. Seventy-three percent of the subjects studied indicated the presence of emotional problems. Thus the data from this study indeed support the researcher's belief that epileptic children need health care which is capable of assessing and meeting a broad spectrum of needs. Developmental delays and poor self-concept are but two of a myriad of possible problems.

The concept of control can have a significant role in the formations of children's self-concept. As discussed in the theoretical framework, children are concerned, from the toddler stage on, with mastery and control of themselves and their environment. It is possible that if epileptics are enabled to feel more in control of themselves and their disease, they may feel better about themselves and thus have a better self-concept.

Other studies have not attempted to link epileptic children's knowledge of their disease with self-concept. However, Long and Moore (1979) did consider self-concept as one of their variables in their study of English families with an epileptic child. These researchers did find that the epileptic children in their study did have a lower self-concept than that of their normal siblings. Frank-Pizzaglia and Pizzaglia (1976) reported that subjects in their study of epileptic children in Cesena, Italy, demonstrated feelings of inferiority and insecurity.

Hodgeman, Iker, McAnarney, McKinney, Myers, Parmalee, Schuster, and Tutihasi (1979) explored the relationship between intelligence level of epileptic children and their self-images. Their hypothesis that higher intelligence would favor a better self-image was not confirmed. The researcher's hypothesis for this study stated that a relationship between school age epileptic children's knowledge of their disease and their self-concept does exist. The work of Hodgeman et al. supports the results of this study and this researcher's hypotheses.

Although the researcher's first hypothesis in this study was significant at the .05 level, there were confounding variables for which there was no inherent control. The level of understanding of the subjects' parents undoubtedly affected the subjects' scores on the knowledge tool. The knowledge tool has not been standardized for different developmental levels. Finally, criteria for scoring the knowledge tool were at best somewhat subjective.

The fact that the researcher's second hypothesis was not supported by the data may indicate problems inherent in the knowledge tool. Whereas the results of the HFDs were scored according to age and predetermined developmental standards, the knowledge tool did not have this capability. A further undesirable characteristic of the knowledge tool was the use of open-ended questions. The open-ended questions provided the opportunity for the children to say they did not know the answer rather than to attempt to answer the questions.

Although the Piers-Harris Self-concept Scale has been found to be reliable, the reading level of the subjects was undoubtedly a confounding variable and thus influenced the final results. Several of the subjects were unable to read the questions on the self-concept scale and required the assistance of the researcher.

Koppitz Evaluation of Children's HFDs appears to have been a reliable method of scoring the children's drawings. The criteria are straightforward and developmentally delineated. There were instances, however, when the researcher should have been more detailed in validating with the children the different parts of their drawings.

Points related to Excerpt 8-4 for consideration in understanding interpretations and discussions include the following.

1. It is important to have an introduction to orient the reader to the content that follows. Writing an introduction is often difficult for students because they believe it to be redundant. The introduction is typically written after the content has been described.

2. The author wrote that a negative correlation was "proven." Kerlinger (1964) wrote

   Let us flatly assert that nothing can be 'proved' scientifically. All one can do is to bring evidence to bear that such-and-such a proposition is true. . . . Thus the interpretation of the analysis of research data can never use the term proof in the logical sense of the word. Interpretation, rather, must concern itself with the evidence for or against the validity of tested hypotheses. (pp. 621–623)

3. In the third paragraph, the author expounded upon the importance of these children being oriented to their disease. Some critics would suggest that the author went too far because her study does not investigate educational *techniques*. The author only investigated *knowledge*, not *how* it was acquired. On the contrary, the inclusion of ramifications as presented is proper because nurses should be guided in using research findings whenever they might be appropriately applied. To be logical, the author could have noted that she was diverging from a discussion related strictly and unswervingly to the data.

4. Is there a logical leap in the fourth paragraph from self-concept to emotional problem? The concepts are related and the missing bridge may be in the conceptual framework the author used or in what the tools were designed to measure. Likewise, the term "development delays" does not fit with the material in the excerpt.

5. In the fifth paragraph, the author ties her findings in with her theoretical framework. The implied theoretical framework is developmental, but it is not identified as such or referenced in the excerpt.

6. Relationship to specific studies reviewed is given. It seems a little confusing to state the hypothesis of a relationship existing and not clarify that the relationship is a negative one as compared with Hodgeman, et al., who *failed to confirm* their hypothesis. Therefore, can the Hodgeman, et al., findings logically be said to support the author's hypothesis?

7. The plural "hypotheses" may be used inappropriately in some cases in this discussion because only one of the author's hypotheses was statistically significant.

8. Note that the author points out possible questions of validity of even her significant findings.

9. An evaluation of each of the research tools is presented.

WRITING THE SUMMARY OF THE RESEARCH STUDY

Following the details of the presentation and analysis of the data, the interpretation and discussion of the findings, a summary of the study is indicated. The summary should be about one double-spaced typewritten page; that is, it should be brief. The purpose of the study should be the beginning of the summary; the conceptual framework should be identified, as well as the research design and the tools used for data collection. Whether to include the review of the literature in the summary is questionable. Fox (1982) indicated, "The review of the literature, description of the sample, and description of the instruments are all omitted or treated extremely briefly" (p. 440). Another researcher once told me that the answer to every question about research is, "It depends. . . ." That answer certainly applies to the question of what should be included in the summary of a research report. It might be helpful to consider the purpose of the summary. The summary may be the only part that some reviewers will read. It will be the first part many more will read, and they will look for the other parts depending on what you include in your summary. If the most outstanding feature about your study is the population you sampled, a mention of the population should be included in your summary. If your study clearly supports or refutes some well-known work, that fact and the identification of the salient work should be included. As a rule, you do not include the findings in the summary because you are going to draw conclusions in the next section and those conclusions will be based on the findings.

Good and Scates (1954) pointed out that the summary "is not the place for the introduction of new data or for encyclopedic enumeration of details reported earlier in the manuscript, but for final synthesis of the whole study" (p. 851). Perhaps Meyer and Heidgerken's (1962) description of the summary will help put it in perspective: "The summary is offered to preface the conclusions as a brief reference relating the means to the end" (p. 416). Two examples of summaries presented below are from master's theses and represent the summary of a descriptive study (Excerpt 8-5) and the summary of a quasiexperimental study (Excerpt 8-6).

EXCERPT 8-5

LOCUS OF CONTROL AND SUCCESSFUL WEIGHT LOSS

SUMMARY

To study the relationship between locus of control and successful weight loss, the researcher conducted a correlational study.

The convenience sample was 21 women enrolled in a continuing education course, "The Psychology of Losing Weight and Never Finding It Again." At a regularly scheduled meeting of the group, selected demographic data were obtained, weights were recorded, and locus of control was measured with the Adult Nowicki-Strickland Internal-External Control Scale. At the completion of the 6-week behavioral course presenting the components of contextual shift, the subjects were weighed and again completed the Adult Nowicki-Strickland Internal-External Control Scale. The data were then analyzed.

EXCERPT 8-6

EFFECTS OF GROUP AND INDIVIDUAL PRE-PTCA TEACHING ON ANXIETY LEVEL AND KNOWLEDGE GAIN IN CARDIOVASCULAR CLIENTS

SUMMARY

A quasiexperimental study was conducted to investigate the differential effects of teaching methods (group and individual) and the presence or absence of the family members, on the knowledge gain and anxiety of PTCA subjects after client teaching. The subjects were 21 PTCA clients admitted to an acute care, general referral and teaching hospital in a large metropolitan area in the southeast. All subjects received structured teaching consisting of an angioplasty education booklet and a discussion session with the researcher. Group teaching was used when two or more subjects were on the same floor. Individual teaching was used when only one subject was on a unit. Each subject completed a knowledge questionnaire developed by the researcher and the STAI state anxiety inventory prior to reading the booklet and again several hours later after the discussion teaching session with the researcher. Family members were included in the teaching when they were available.

Your first question may be the identification of PTCA. It is the abbreviation for *percutaneous transluminal coronary angioplasty* which is an alternative to coronary artery bypass graft surgery. This abbreviation is a good example of how much the researcher must define the terms in order to communicate. The problem with the abbreviation is that the researcher believed that the name of the procedure was no more illuminating than the abbreviation, and anyone interested in reading about the procedure would recognize the abbreviation. You might have a similar problem with the term *locus of control* in the first summary. If you are interested in that construct, you will be informed after reading the summary. Otherwise, you may not know what to expect. Other points to be observed in Excerpts 8-5 and 8-6 are listed below.

1. Both are short, well within the suggested one page guideline.
2. Both present the purpose of the study in the first sentence.
3. Both identify the sample and give clear indications of how the samples were obtained.
4. Both researchers identify the type of research design used.
5. Both summaries contain the names of the research tools that were employed in the data collection.

6. The time frame of the study is clear in both summaries.

7. In Excerpt 8-5, it is not informative to read that the data were analyzed. That sentence could be omitted without reducing the information contained in the summary.

8. In Excerpt 8-6 the STAI refers to the State Trait Anxiety Inventory. It is not clear why both the abbreviation and the name were needed or, if both were going to be presented, why "trait" was omitted from the name. While this and many of the other comments seem unduly "picayune," the goal is to be as precise as possible.

9. Neither researcher included conceptual framework, literature review, or findings in the summary. As you know from the discussion above, the conceptual framework should be identified, but it is not necessary and, in most cases, not desirable to include the literature review or findings.

CONCLUSIONS

At this point, you must make some concluding statements about your study. Conclusions should be based on the findings, which were based on the hypotheses. Remember there are no surprises. The conclusions should emerge gracefully from all that has preceded. "The conclusion comprises the outcome of the total study. It stipulates whether or not the specific purpose has been served. It may provide the answer to the problem. It is offered in reference to both the logical hypothesis and the empiric test" (Meyer and Heidgerken 1962, p. 416). Further points about conclusions can be made with reference to the conclusions that followed the summaries presented in Excerpts 8-5 and 8-6.

EXCERPT 8-7

LOCUS OF CONTROL AND SUCCESSFUL WEIGHT LOSS

(From same thesis as Excerpt 8-5)

CONCLUSIONS

Although not statistically significant, the findings are noteworthy:

1. Those who lost the most weight were more internally controlled when tested at the first group session.

2. Those who lost the most weight changed more toward the direction of internality.

EXCERPT 8-8

EFFECTS OF GROUP AND INDIVIDUAL PRE-PTCA TEACHING ON ANXIETY LEVEL AND KNOWLEDGE GAIN IN CARDIOVASCULAR CLIENTS

(From same thesis as Excerpt 8-6)

CONCLUSIONS

Based on the data and findings, the following conclusions seem warranted:

1. That group and individual client teaching are equally effective methods of improving client knowledge.
2. That group and individual client teaching are equally effective methods of altering client anxiety (although a trend was noted for group teaching to be more effective).
3. That the inclusion of family members in client education does not significantly alter the knowledge gain or anxiety of subjects, and may hinder client learning in certain circumstances.
4. That overall PTCA client education using a booklet and discussion session significantly improves client knowledge about the PTCA procedure, and pre- and post-procedure care.
5. That overall PTCA client education using a booklet and discussion has no effect on altering client anxiety.

The following comments are offered to sharpen your understanding of and familiarity with conclusions.

1. Conclusions are usually listed, as in the two examples presented.
2. The list of conclusions is introduced by a statement such as the ones presented in the excerpts. Excerpt 8-7 is confusing because the researcher does not make it clear that the conclusions are *based* on the findings. The *findings* in this case were: the mean weight loss for subjects internally controlled was 9.75 pounds compared to the mean weight loss of 5.27 pounds for the externally controlled group; the correlation between weight loss and locus of control change in the direction of internally was not significant ($r = .145$, $p = .265$). Findings are the facts as you obtained them; conclusions are what you make of the findings.
3. The degree to which you can generalize in your conclusion is limited by your sampling techniques. If you randomly sampled from a popu-

lation, you can generalize to that population. If you used a convenience sample, you can make your conclusions for *that sample only.*

4. If you have questions about the validity of the conclusions drawn for a study, go back to the presentation and analysis of the data and draw your own conclusions. Give yourself credit; you are an intelligent person, and you can make your own decisions about whether reported findings are useful for your purposes.

5. There is also the controversial question of whether you can draw conclusions about nonsignificant findings. When you see the $p = .265$ as the basis for the second conclusion in Excerpt 8-7, do you agree with the researcher? Statisticians would usually say unequivocally that no conclusion could be drawn, and strictly speaking, that is true. What if the probability had been .06? The point of reporting is to communicate. It is mandatory to communicate accurately. Do you have some responsibility for communicating the direction of the data, however insignificant? The safe practice is to present the facts and what conclusions *you* are drawing from those facts. The reader is expected to use the information intelligently and responsibly.

6. Conclusions are written in the present tense because it is assumed that they are not limited to a specific time period.

7. It may be picayune, but Excerpt 8-8 would be enhanced by omitting "That" from the beginning of each conclusion.

The conclusions lead logically to a set of recommendations. Perhaps Meyer and Heidgerken (1962) expressed it best:

> It must be remembered that research moves slowly. It advances by inches rather than by tremendous leaps. . . . Thus, each step in the total process may be considered for its own sake and with regard to its place in the complete study. All studies are useful, even if they only contribute the suggestion of an erroneous course of action. . . . A researcher often must proceed step by step or inch by inch toward a positive and over-all contribution to knowledge. (p. 415)

RECOMMENDATIONS

Research usually generates more questions than it answers. It is the responsibility of the researcher to make recommendations that provide directions for future investigators in seeking answers to the new questions raised. Another responsibility lies in the application of the research findings to nursing practice (or education or administration as indicated). The recommendations should be based on the findings and the conclusions. The recommendations do not reflect some extraneous thoughts the researcher might have had about another unrelated problem. One of the best sources for ideas for a research topic is the recommendations made in previous studies. Consider Excerpts 8-9 and 8-10 for additional familiarity with the recommendations section.

EXCERPT 8-9

LOCUS OF CONTROL AND SUCCESSFUL WEIGHT LOSS

(From same thesis as Excerpts 8-5 and 8-7)

RECOMMENDATIONS

Based on the data and conclusions, the investigator offers the following recommendations for further research:

1. Further investigation should be conducted with randomized sampling to control extraneous variables.
2. A more specific scale for measuring weight locus of control should be used.
3. Nurses should explore the implication of the concept of locus of control in therapeutic interventions with clients.

Recommendations for nursing practice include the following:

1. Nurses should make interventions relevant to clients' locus of control to provide more effective nursing care.
2. Nurses should consider the role of assisting the client to lose weight, a requirement for health maintenance and prevention of illness.

EXCERPT 8-10

EFFECTS OF GROUP AND INDIVIDUAL PRE-PTCA TEACHING ON ANXIETY LEVEL AND KNOWLEDGE GAIN IN CARDIOVASCULAR CLIENTS

(From same thesis as Excerpts 8-6 and 8-8)

RECOMMENDATIONS

Based on the data and conclusions, the investigator offers the following recommendations for further research:

1. That further investigations of this type be conducted with a larger sample size and random sampling, to permit generalization of the results.

2. That further investigations be conducted where the client educators are the staff nurses who routinely do the teaching so that the results are reflective of the actual hospital setting.

3. That further investigations be conducted that
   a. examine client anxiety the morning after teaching and before a PTCA procedure, and
   b. examine client ability to apply the teaching information appropriately before, during, and after a procedure.

4. That further studies be conducted which investigate the influence of the presence of family members on adult client education.

5. That group teaching be utilized in nursing practice as an effective and efficient method of client education.

IMPLICATIONS OF NURSING PRACTICE

The results of this study have several implications for nursing practice which relate to the areas of research outlined by Redman (1971). Group education should be used in practice as an effective and efficient method of client teaching as well as help contain the costs of professional services. Client education booklets (as the angioplasty booklet) should be developed, evaluated, and used in nursing practice as primary teaching tools. If future studies indicate that client teaching does not alter anxiety, nursing practice should implement new interventions to decrease anxiety, especially in cardiovascular clients. Finally, since the results of this and previous studies ... are inconclusive, nursing practice should determine how to use the family in client education and care.

You probably have already identified several points about these excerpts. The following comments may augment your own thoughts.

1. Both recommendations indicated that they were based on the data and conclusions. It might be preferable to indicate that the recommendations are based on the *findings* and conclusions simply because findings seems to be a broader term and would include data. This point is not worth arguing about, as it is strictly a matter of preference and rationale. You will soon notice that every research teacher or thesis adviser has certain preferred or favorite ways of expressing a particular entity.

2. Although both researchers offer recommendations for further research and further practice, Excerpt 8-10 presents the practice recommendations in paragraph, rather than list, form. Again, the form is a matter of preference. Lists make the points more emphatically while paragraphs allow you to provide greater discussion and connection of ideas.

3. It is customary to suggest that the study be repeated with modifications as appropriate. *Replication* means that the study is done again exactly as it was originally. Often replication is suggested with the setting or population being different. In general, if the results were significant in the direction hypothesized, replication is indicated to confirm the findings; replication on a different population is indicated to generalize the findings. If the results were not significant, the recommendations will probably suggest changes in one or more of the following: the tools used for the data collection, a larger sample size (frequently suggested but be reasonable; if the original sample was quite adequate, there is some other weakness), or a tighter design (meaning better control of the variables).

4. Since the data from the two studies from which Excerpts 8-9 and 8-10 were taken are not available, a judgment as to whether the recommendations are related is impossible. The conclusions, however, are presented and the second recommendation for practice in Excerpt 8-9 does not appear to be directly related to the conclusions. We might wonder if the recommendation is related to the findings since the conclusions should reflect the findings. There is a great temptation to use the recommendations to make a plea for one's favorite cause. The temptation should be avoided by sticking to the logic of the research process and addressing only those issues related to the research done. There are other opportunities to do other studies and write other papers. Avoid trying to put everything into one.

Writing the recommendations is often the last act of the research process. As such, it is often done in haste because time is running (or has run) out. Recommendations require thought and should not be just the routine replication suggestion. "Therefore, the final word of advice is to exert every effort in the planning of research to allow sufficient time for the proper preparation of the research report" (Fox 1982, p. 442). Actually, a final recommendation is that you go and do more nursing research. "Thus, the study ended as it began—on a note from the past and an inquiry for the future" (Meyer and Heidgerken 1962, p. 416).

SUMMARY

This chapter completes Part I, the research process. You have now been through all of the steps involved in initiating, conducting, analyzing, drawing conclusions, and making recommendations. There is more. You must write a research report, for if you never report it, what contribution could your efforts possibly make? Part II is a discussion of writing the research report.

Suggestions for Further Study

The following suggestions are designed to facilitate your practice in "making sense" of data.

1. Review the excerpts presented in Chapter 8 and make comments that were *not included* in the comments that followed each excerpt. For example, following early excerpts, comments were made about problems that also appeared in later excerpts but were ignored in the later ones. You should be able to pick out those areas that could be improved, and you can probably find some that were not suggested.

2. Review the presentation and analysis of data, interpretations (or discussions), summaries, conclusions, and recommendations in at least three articles from nursing research journals. In what ways do they substantiate the points made in Chapter 8? In what ways are they different than was suggested in Chapter 8? How are you going to resolve the differences?

3. Present the findings, discuss the findings, summarize the study, draw conclusions, and make appropriate recommendations for the research project you have been developing.

Suggestions for Additional Reading

Abbott, N. K. "Findings, Conclusions, and Recommendations," in S. D. Krampitz and N. Pavlovich (Eds.), *Readings for Nursing Research.* St. Louis: The C. V. Mosby Company, 1981.

Good, C. V., and Scates, D. E. *Methods of Research: Educational, Psychological, Sociological.* New York: Appleton-Century-Crofts, Inc., 1954.

Kerlinger, F. N. *Foundations of Behavioral Research.* New York: Holt, Rinehart and Winston, Inc., 1964.

Komnenich, P., and Noack, J. A. "The Process of Critiquing," in S. D. Krampitz and N. Pavlovich (Eds.), *Readings for Nursing Research.* St. Louis: The C. V. Mosby Company, 1981.

Meyer, B., and Heidgerken, L. E. *Introduction to Research in Nursing.* Philadelphia: J. B. Lippincott Company, 1962.

Polit, D. F., and Hungler, B. P. *Nursing Research: Principles and Methods* (2nd edition). Philadelphia: J. B. Lippincott Company, 1983.

Publication Manual of the American Psychological Association (3rd edition). Washington, DC: American Psychological Association, 1983.

Wandelt, M. A. *Guide for the Beginning Researcher.* New York: Appleton-Century-Crofts, 1970.

PART II
WRITING THE RESEARCH REPORT

The second part of this book is designed to provide guidelines for writing a research report. One of the most difficult adjustments creative students have to make is to learn to write the facts and eliminate the frills of quotes from Shakespeare and Chaucer, however amusing and interesting those bits of literature may be. The beginning report writer has difficulty defining terms and sticking to those definitions; the tendency is to make the report "interesting" by varying the terms and metaphors. Such literary techniques serve to obscure the precision of the research process and are to be avoided. Another problem causing battles between students and research advisers is over the necessity of rewriting and rewriting and rewriting reports before the final copy is acceptable.

Chapter 9 contains suggestions for effective preparation of the report. Frequently committed errors are included with suggestions for avoiding such mistakes. Examples of well-written reports are presented in contrast to reports that have some identified weaknesses.

Chapter 9
How are you going to tell others about it?

WRITING THE REPORT AND PUBLISHING

Chapter Objectives

Upon successful completion of this chapter the student will be able to

- Describe the purpose of an abstract of a piece of research
- List several places one would look for abstracts for various research topics
- Write a succinct, well-organized abstract that appropriately describes a research project
- Describe the appropriate content for the parts of a research report
- Write a report of a research project

INTRODUCTION

So you have always wanted to be a writer of thrilling literature of mystery and intrigue. Well, now is *not* your chance! Technical writing is serious business. In reporting research, you report concisely but precisely what the purpose of the study was, how you formulated a research question or hypothesis to fulfill that purpose, the conceptual context of your question or hypothesis, what others have done that is related to your purpose, how you collected data in order to test your hypothesis or answer your research question, what you got when you collected your data, how you organized and analyzed your data, and your interpretations of your findings. It is also important for you to relate your findings to the purpose of the study, the conceptual framework, and other related studies. Make recommendations for nursing practice and for further research, when appropriate. The "when appropriate" is emphasized because you must be careful not to recommend something when insufficient data are available to warrant such practice. It is almost always possible and appropriate to make recommendations for further research.

Do not decide at this point that you are tired of the whole project and you do not wish to publish at this time. There are three considerations which should influence you.

1. You have an ethical obligation to communicate your findings to other nurses so that they can benefit from your efforts and build a body of nursing knowledge (more about ethics in Chapter 11). Do not consider your study unimportant if you were careful in your design and data collection and analysis and found anything (even if it was negative). There is a problem of deciding on the best way to communicate. Journals typically run several months to a year behind and have such space limitations that they may not show the enthusiasm that is being suggested about publishing your manuscript. Do not despair—there are a growing number of research symposia all over the country to which you may submit an abstract of your study for consideration for presentation. The outline for the presentation is similar to that for the research process, and you will have an opportunity to discuss your findings and impressions with others interested in your subject. That is fun!

2. If you do not do it *now*, the probability of your doing it later becomes slimmer and slimmer with every passing day. You may take a little recess from your efforts only if you put it on your calendar to do it soon with absolutely no excuses. Not only is it difficult to come back to the

project later, but the world is being denied the information. In addition, someone else may publish a similar study which would influence the editors or the program planning committee to choose the other one over yours.

3. Only after you have published articles and research studies in a specific area, is it likely that you will be successful in applying for funding. Funding agents are prone to support success; that is, they are compelled to support researchers whom they know to have a good chance of producing. It is necessary for the funding agents to maintain this approach no matter how unfair it may seem to beginning researchers. The reason is clear if you think about it—they want to show results also. The best way to do so is to go with those researchers and institutions who have produced in the past. For that reason you may have to do a couple or more studies on your own time and at your own expense in order to demonstrate your sincerity and research competence.

THE TEN COMMANDMENTS OF WRITING

Editors tell us that they have great difficulty getting manuscripts into forms that are publishable. The following points are frequently made:

1. Thou shalt not use a big word when a smaller word will do.

2. Thou shalt not keep the reader in suspense. Say what you are going to say up front. If the reader is interested, the remainder of the manuscript will be read; if not, the reader has not wasted time on something that is outside immediate interests.

3. Thou shalt not use more space than is absolutely necessary. Space costs money; therefore, publishers want articles as concise as possible.

4. Thou shalt not split infinitives or dangle participles. These errors are common and unnecessary. Go back to a basic English text and review as necessary. If you do not know what an infinitive or a participle is (and graduate students have denied any knowledge of such), it is time to learn. Take a continuing education course in technical writing or perhaps even a course for credit. Do not be embarrassed about not knowing—acknowledge your deficiencies and do something about it. Some of the most heated arguments among university faculty have been over the application of rules of English composition.

5. Thou shalt not write without an outline. Do not subject readers (even teachers) to a potpourri of words. You and your readers will proceed more efficiently if you organize your thoughts in a logical order to accomplish your purpose or communicate your message.

6. Thou shalt not write without a message. You do not just report data—you report data in order to make some statement about a problem, a theory, or other research. As you write keep in mind constantly what the theme of your communication is. What is the "bottom line"? What is the point?

7. Thou shalt not make unsupported value judgments in your writing. Do not attack someone or something as "bad" or "inadequate." Be objective in critiques: state what is included, what seems to be missing, leaps in logic that you have difficulty making, and inconsistencies. To mention that an article is inconsistent is certainly a value judgment, but it is more informative when supported with an example than saying that the report was "poor." Perhaps the problem with value judgments (positive as well as negative) is that they do not communicate anything and only create a feeling for or against the study. Just because one has been told that the study is "good" does not necessarily indicate that one should read or replicate the study; likewise, if a study is "bad" it may be that the data are inappropriately analyzed, but the review of the literature may be just what the reviewer has been searching for.

8. Thou shalt not omit a reference. The crime of plagiarism is serious and inexcusable. It seems so easy to simply give credit where credit is due. Rarely do two individuals express ideas alike. So express the idea your way, reference the source of the idea, and everyone has gained. The previous author gets exposure and credit; you gain authority for your statement since it is backed by someone else, or at least related to some other authority. The better known the authority, the more weight your statement will have until you become the authority by your research findings.

9. Thou shalt not hesitate to seek help appropriately as needed. Do not believe that any question is too trivial or that you will appear less sophisticated than you wish to appear if you ask about something you do not know. On the other hand, do not waste the time and impose on the good nature of busy people by "bugging" them with questions you could more easily find answers to in the library or some other readily available resource. Learn to utilize all of the resources available to you—library materials, government agencies and publica-

tions, clinical settings, and people who might be called experts on certain topics. Researchers usually are delighted to talk with you about what they are doing. The closer your research is to theirs, the more interested they will be in your ideas. In fact, many researchers are starved for someone to listen to them and may welcome you.

10. Thou shalt not become discouraged. If you are going to do research and publish, you will become "public." You will be criticized. Others will make suggestions, offer support, or tear your ideas apart. Do not be surprised. Do not take it personally. There are manuscripts for master's theses in drawers of faculty and students who will never receive the degree they have almost earned. They, unfortunately, were not willing to respond to critiques offered by faculty and make sometimes simple modifications so that the theses could meet the requirements. Whether the faculty criticisms were warranted is beside the point—the fact is that funding agencies, faculty, editors, and research review committees have a certain amount of authority and thus control. If you recognize that and can adjust to it, you can publish your studies. If you become angry and possessive of your work, you may have difficulty making your findings known. Rarely, if ever, is anything submitted anywhere without having some editorial changes made. The way to learn to write is similar to learning to play tennis, or swim, or ride a bicycle—you practice. Writing may never become easy for you, but you can become more successful at it. It can be rewarding.

ABSTRACTS

When you decide to submit your study for publication or to present it to a group of peers at a research symposium, you will usually be asked to submit an abstract. An abstract is a summary of your research. The length of the abstract may be limited to 250 to 500 words. Some limitations are as severe as 50 words and others are as generous as 1,000 words. You must know (and adhere to) the requirements of the journal or committee to which you are submitting your abstract. For journals, the information is usually in one of the first few pages of the journal. The "call for papers" from the symposium committee usually indicates the desired length of the abstract. Also there may be guidelines specifying what the abstract should contain.

If the instructions regarding the abstract are not clear, the following suggestions may be considered (see *Publication Manual of the American Psychological Association,* 1983):

1. The abstract is used by some reference sources to index and retrieve information; therefore, the abstract should be self-contained and clear, without having to refer to the body of the paper.

2. Limit the abstract to 100 to 200 words.

3. Include statements of the problems, the conceptual framework, and methodology (description of subjects, research design, tools, and data-gathering procedures).

4. The abstract should reflect the importance of various parts in the body of the paper.

5. Summarize findings, including any statistical significance levels and conclusions drawn.

6. Include the name, title, and institution of the author and the title of the paper so that the abstract can stand alone and be readily identified.

7. Double-space unless instructions specify otherwise.

Examples and Critiques of Abstracts of Nursing Research

Rarely are there perfect specimens of research or abstracts. In the spirit of constructive critique and learning, read the following abstract and evaluate it according to the criteria given above and according to the Ten Commandments of Writing.

EXCERPT 9-1 _____

RELATIONSHIP OF SOCIAL SKILLS TRAINING FOR CHRONIC
SCHIZOPHRENICS IN BOARDING HOMES AND THEIR
ADJUSTMENT IN THE COMMUNITY

by
Jane Doe
Staff Development Coordinator
State Hospital

ABSTRACT

Caring for the chronically mentally ill has historically proved to be a difficult task. Concerns as to how to best meet their needs with limited finances has created a cyclic migration from the community to large state hospitals and back to the community. None of these attempts has made any impact in treating these individuals. Presently residing in the community after years of institutionalization, these individuals lack the resources needed to adapt to their environment. A review of studies dealing with the effects of treatment for the chronically mentally ill revealed that individual therapy, group therapy, work therapy, and drug therapy did not alter community functioning. This researcher believed that a social skills group for this targeted population would supplement their limited resources and facilitate their adjustment in the community.

To determine if chronic schizophrenic clients who received social skills training would show a greater increase in community adjustment than a control group receiving outpatient treatment, the researcher undertook a quasi experimental, test-retest design. The ten subjects were English speaking male and female chronic schizophrenic clients, ages 23 to 47, living in boarding homes in an urban setting. Five of these individuals from the same boarding home participated in an eight week social skills group. All ten of the subjects were given the Bell Adjustment Inventory before and after the group. Differences in scores on adjustment between the experimental and control groups were compared utilizing the Mann-Whitney U Test. Analysis of the data revealed a significant difference between these two groups when assessed for level of adjustment. The results of the study support the researcher's hypothesis that clients would show an increase in the level of community adjustment after experience in a social skills group as compared to a control group receiving routine outpatient treatment.

This abstract does have a title, the name of the author and her position and institution are indicated. Assume it was double-spaced, what about the length? It is too long, containing more than the desirable 200 words. (To estimate the number of words contained in a passage, count the number of lines, multiply by the number of spaces per line, and divide by five.) This abstract is self-contained, for it is complete without referring to the body of the paper. Consider the first sentence. What does it tell you the paper is about? Nothing—related perhaps to chronically mentally ill something. This wording problem also appears in the title. The acceptable usage is to provide nouns rather than have the modifiers standing alone; that is, "mentally ill. . . ." The noun is missing. It would be better to indicate chronically mentally ill individuals, or more specifically adults.

Can you find the split infinitive in the second sentence? "To best meet" is the error. Note that so far it is unclear who is concerned or who is trying to meet the needs—what needs? Meeting needs with limited finances is rarely a good idea; the implied meaning while probably not particularly confusing is not well stated. Why "large" state hospitals? Is there something about large that the reader is supposed to know? Are small state hospitals doing something better? Are there any small state hospitals? Why are private hospitals different? Again, the implication is that large state hospitals are the focus of the study, but that is not stated.

In sentence three—what attempts? So far, the author has mentioned caring and concerns. Is the reader to infer some sort of attempts from that? At least individuals have been recognized; that is, a noun has now been included. Notice the "impact on treating." Is that where you would desire the impact? Impact on behavior or adjustment or some other outcome would seem more appropriate.

"Presently residing in the community after years of institutionalization, these individuals lack the resources needed to adapt to their environment." This sentence is inconsistent with the second sentence which had them cycling between those large state hospitals and the community.

The following sentence refers to the review of the literature and yet the focus of the study has not been stated. Even so, there is a list of therapies which do not alter community functioning. What is the problem with the community functioning? What alterations are desired in functioning of the community?

The last sentence in the first paragraph indicates the researcher believes that a social skills group would supplement limited resources. It was just noted in the previous sentence, however, that group therapy does not alter community functioning. Is there a relationship between community functioning and limited resources? What, if anything, is different about group therapy and social skills groups?

The first sentence in paragraph two is redundant, as it repeats much of what was in the previous sentence. With only ten subjects, it would be helpful to know how many were male and how many female. For such a small number, there is a wide age range, and not much information is given about the boarding homes, except that they are in an urban setting.

In the next two sentences, the five subjects in one boarding home participated in an eight-week social skill group. Was this group the experimental group? What does the author mean by "given the Bell Adjustment Inventory before and after the group"? It probably does not mean before and after each group session, but instead refers to prior to the beginning of the series of sessions and after the termination of the series.

"Differences in scores on adjustment between the experimental and control groups were compared utilizing the Mann-Whitney U Test." What exactly is compared is not clear. It is most likely that each subject served as his or her own control, with the difference noted between the score obtained on the test the first time it was administered and the second. The experimental group's difference scores were probably compared to the control group's difference scores. Another noteworthy observation in the sentence under consideration is the use of the word "utilizing" when "using" would have done just as well. The next sentence indicates that the analysis was significant, but does not give the level of significance.

The last sentence could be improved by omitting the words "would show an." The sentence would then be: "The results of the study support the researcher hypothesis that clients increase in the level of community adjustment after experience in a social skills group as compared to a control group receiving routine outpatient treatment." Note that the possessive on the word "researcher's" was also dropped. What does this statement imply as far as the generalizability of this study? That is not clear, and it may be appropriately left to the reader to draw conclusions. Other critics would argue that the researcher has a responsibility to make a statement regarding the population to which the study can be generalized. Given significant results as reported in the abstract, the researcher should consider implications for practice and make recommendations for further research.

It cannot be overemphasized that each critic or reviewer will have a unique opinion. Researchers, particularly new researchers, must accept the fact that improvement is always possible, and there are always those individuals who are ready to criticize. Students argue that if they could take an "incomplete" in a course they could write a proposal that would not have to be revised. There are a couple of problems with that position: (1) It is unlikely that a student or anyone can produce the "perfect" product that needs no revisions. (2) The "real world" does not often operate in such a way as to provide unlimited or even "enough" time to do the caliber of job one would like to do; there are always deadlines for manuscripts, grant proposals, fiscal years, academic terms, and one's own priorities.

Learn to listen to criticism. Let the information sit in your mind until you have a chance to consider it objectively. Accept what makes sense, get additional opinions on what does not, and make the changes that you can and wish to make. An improved version of the abstract critiqued follows.

EXCERPT 9-2

COMMUNITY ADJUSTMENT FOLLOWING SOCIAL SKILLS
TRAINING OF
INDIVIDUALS DIAGNOSED AS CHRONIC SCHIZOPHRENICS
AND LIVING IN BOARDING HOMES

by
Jane Doe
State Development Coordinator
State Hospital

ABSTRACT

The purpose of this study was to determine if a social skills training group experience would increase the community adjustment of individuals who were living in boarding homes and diagnosed as chronic schizophrenics. A test-retest quasi-experimental design was implemented. Ten subjects made up the convenience sample of volunteers from two boarding homes in the same general community. The five subjects in the experimental group were from the same boarding home and participated in an eight-week social skills group. The control group consisted of individuals from the other boarding home. The control group received routine outpatient treatment. Characteristics of the subjects included: males and females, ages 23 to 47, and English speaking. The Bell Adjustment Inventory was administered to all 10 subjects prior to the first social skills group meeting and after the completion of the series of eight meetings. The pre-post difference scores of the experimental group were significantly greater than the difference scores of the control group. Application of the Mann-Whitney U Test yielded a difference at the .05 level of significance. Although generalization of these results is inappropriate due to the nonrandomness of the sample and the circumscribed population, replication and consideration of other studies to investigate ways of enhancing the quality of life of individuals with major psychiatric diagnoses are recommended.

You should be able to improve even on this version. For a start, the theoretical framework is not explicit and the abstract borders on being too long. What are some other criticisms? Rewrite the abstract improving on the ones reviewed.

Another example of an abstract submitted for consideration for presentation at a regional research symposium follows.

EXCERPT 9-3

THE RELATIONSHIP BETWEEN STAFFING PATTERNS AND
ACCURACY OF
INTAKE AND OUTPUT RECORDING

by
John Doe
City Hospital

ABSTRACT

In order to determine if the type of nursing personnel monitoring intake and output records was a possible contributing factor to inaccurate intake and output records, a descriptive correlational study was conducted. Subjects were 25 patients in the surgical intensive care unit where only registered nurses monitor intake and output, and 25 patients on a general nursing unit where a variety of nursing personnel, including registered nurses, licensed practical nurses, nursing assistants, and students monitor intake and output records.

Each subject was weighed on two consecutive mornings and the weight difference was calculated. The intake and output data were collected from the chart for the 24-hour period between weight determinations. A difference was then calculated between the intake and output for each subject. The weight difference and the intake and output difference were then compared for accuracy. According to definition, accuracy existed when the two differences were in the same direction of gain or loss.

Data were then collected on the nursing personnel staffing in each patient care area. Data included age, sex, educational preparation, number of years in nursing, and number of years employed at the institution where the study was performed. These data were then compared between the two nursing groups.

Results from the intake and output data were as follows:

TABLE 1
Accuracy and Inaccuracy of the Intake and
Output Records in the SICU and the GNU

	SURGICAL INTENSIVE CARE UNIT RN STAFFING		GENERAL NURSING UNIT VARIETY OF PERSONNEL	
Accurate	84%	(n=21)	32%	(n=8)
Inaccurate	16%	(n=4)	68%	(n=17)

166

CONCLUSIONS

A z test was employed to test the significance of the difference between the intake and output records in each group of subjects. The results obtained were statistically significant at the .05 level. A correlation coefficient between the net difference in weight and the net difference in intake and output for each group was also calculated. The correlation coefficient for the surgical intensive care unit was .77 and statistically significant at the .001 level. The correlation coefficient for the general nursing unit was not statistically significant. Based on the statistical analysis, the null hypothesis of no difference in intake and output accuracy between the two groups was rejected.

This abstract is too long, and rarely is there an opportunity to include a table. The title does not seem to reflect accurately the contents of the abstract. By staffing patterns one might assume how many personnel are on duty, hours worked, or some other form of pattern. This abstract appears to relate more to a study of types of personnel, or types of nursing personnel, or levels of nursing personnel, or preparation of nursing staff as a factor in accuracy of measurement of intake and output. An early question is how the researcher defined intake and output. As one looks over the abstract in order to determine how this dependent variable is being measured, it becomes apparent that the chart is the source of this information. Facetiously, you might question how you measure intake and output from a chart. Seriously, these terms are not defined and the criteria for charting this information are not given. You may think you know what intake and output are, but look at the findings. The surgical intensive care staff were much more accurate than the general nursing unit staff. You should wonder how many of the intensive care patients had indwelling urethral catheters and were being hydrated by intravenous fluids. How much easier and more accurate is it to measure the fluid input and output of patients with catheters and intravenous input than to try to keep an account of what a general unit patient drinks and how much such patients void during a 24-hour period? It is quite possible that some of these variables were controlled, but the reader has no way of knowing that.

More positively, the researcher's method of determining accuracy of measurement was interesting. It seems to make sense but does not reflect the degree of agreement between intake and output and weight. For example, according to the abstract, a patient whose record indicated that he weighed 168 pounds the first morning and 168.2 pounds the second morning with an intake of 3000 cubic centimeters (cc) and an output of 100 cc would be counted as "accurate." A patient who weighed 120 pounds on the first day and 119.9 pounds on the second day and had an input of 1000 cc and an output of 1100 cc would be said to have an "inaccurate" recording. In addition, no information is given about the standardization of the weights—were the patients weighed on the same scales or scales carefully calibrated for accuracy? Are you willing to base nursing practice on such evidence?

These last few comments may be more critical of the design than of the abstract, or the problem is that the abstract does not clearly reflect the study. Further criticism of the information in the abstract, which may reflect the problems with the study, includes the analysis of the data. It is not clear why a z test was chosen for the analysis of the data. The data are frequency data and a Fisher's Exact Test would be helpful in determining differences. The test used to determine the correlation coefficient between the net difference of the intake and output and of the weight is not specified. Again, the fact that the correlation was significant on the surgical intensive care unit and not on the general nursing unit may reflect the difficulty in obtaining accurate information from the charts of the patients on the general nursing unit. Another point you might consider is the importance of obtaining accurate information on the different groups of patients. Accurate intake and output may be extremely important on the surgical intensive care unit, but not of such concern for all patients on the general nursing unit. Patients hospitalized for diagnostic tests or patients ready to be discharged would not necessarily require accurate recordings on intake and output and, therefore, might not get it. It may even be appropriate for the staff to concentrate on items of higher priority.

As a nurse, what implications do you get from this abstract? Should only registered nurses be hired to staff patient care units? Should only nurses (RNs) be assessing intakes and outputs? Should staff development programs for teaching accurate ways of measuring intake and output be initiated in the hospital in which this study was done? Would you do a follow-up study to clarify some of the questions in this research? If so, what problems would you address and how would you address them?

Since the weaknesses of this study seem to be in the design of the study or in the questions about the design, no attempt will be made to rewrite this abstract. To formulate a reasonable version would require a great deal of speculation. In terms of writing style, note the overuse of the term "then" and the wordiness of the last paragraph. The same information could be given as follows:

Using a z test, the difference between the intake and output records of each group of subjects was significant at the .05 level. The correlation coefficient between the net difference in weight and the net difference in intake and output was .77 ($p < .001$) for the surgical intensive care unit and not significant for the general nursing unit. Based on the findings of this study, the null hypothesis of no difference between intake and output records of the patients on the two units was rejected.

BODY OF REPORT

The body of the research report follows the research process outline including the statement of the problem, the theoretical framework, review of literature, research methodology, presentation and analysis of data, discussion of data, conclusions, and recommendations. Notice that the section "summary of the study" has been omitted. The omission is because the "abstract" serves as a summary for reports and, therefore, a summary section is redundant.

The report for publication as a journal article is typically shorter than a thesis or dissertation or project report to a funding agency. The content is reduced by sticking strictly to the message that you wish to convey to the reader, without including all of the important but unnecessary descriptions and rationalizations. You really only need to give the main points because the really interested reader will write to you for more information. A master's thesis may be of any length, but following the outline in this text, they usually run about 50 to 80 pages long. A typical manuscript submitted for publication should be between 15 and 20 pages long (or as specified in the guidelines from the publication to which it is being submitted).

Nursing research journals are excellent sources of research reports. To publish a report here would merely duplicate what is or should be available in the nearest library if not in your own personal library. Read the reports critically and do not hesitate to consider how you might improve upon them.

LIST OF REFERENCES

The list of references at the end of your report is just what the title indicates—a list of the sources to which you referred. The reference list is *not* a list of all the sources you consulted no matter how much you want everyone to know how hard you worked. The purpose is to communicate—you communicate the sources that you used in the preparation of the report. The reference list for an article for publication will most likely be much shorter than the reference list for a thesis.

The form of the entries for the reference list must be consistent with the guidelines you use for writing the report. In the absence of other instructions, the third edition of the *Publication Manual of the American Psychological Association* (1983) is recommended. These guidelines are simple and used by many publishers.

SUMMARY

The research process is not complete until the project has been reported. There are several ways of doing the communication: presentation to peers in classrooms or seminars, regional or broader symposia, written reports for class, theses or dissertations, project reports to sponsoring agencies, or articles written for publication. The outline is similar in each case and follows the research process, usually preceded by an abstract. The content depends on the purpose of the report—to document the entire project or communicate findings with potential for nursing care. Communication should be clear and straightforward in all instances. All references should be accurately documented using an acceptable style for citations.

As you share your report with others, you will be subjected to critique (even if only by the one person who made the initial assignment). Part III of this text follows and includes Chapter 10, a discussion of the purposes and guidelines for appropriate critiquing of nursing research.

Suggestions for Further Study

1. Write a report of the project you have completed. Share the report with your peers.

2. Discuss with your research advisor whether you should submit your report for consideration for publication or for presentation at a symposium. Get clarification as to why the report should be shared with others or what it would take to make it of a caliber that could be shared. What are some reasons for not sharing a report at a given time?

3. Evaluate your project on the basis of what you would do differently if you (a) could start over but still had the same time and resources limitations; (b) had more time; (c) had more resources (make a wish list of what you would like to have); and (d) had had more knowledge at the time you began.

4. Read at least two research articles in areas that interest you. The authors of the articles obviously had something they wanted to communicate—you can help by being a "consumer."

Suggestions for Additional Reading

Publication Manual of the American Psychological Association (3rd edition). Washington, DC: American Psychology Association, 1983.

Rodale, J. I. *The Synonym Finder.* Emmaus, PA: Rodale Press, 1978.

Strunk, W., and White, E. B. *The Elements of Style* (3rd edition). New York: Macmillan Publishing Company, Inc., 1979.

PART III
CRITIQUING NURSING RESEARCH

The third part of this book is designed to sharpen the awareness of nurses of the quality and value of research and related literature. There has been a tendency among students and graduates to believe anything that is in print. It is truly easier to accept on faith that which we read. It is also dangerous, unethical, and irresponsible to do so. The purpose of critique is not to denigrate the work of another; the purpose is to identify strengths, build on those strengths, and contribute to the science of nursing. Obviously, weaknesses are also identified so that the work is put in proper perspective and shortcomings reduced or eliminated.

Chapter 10 discusses guidelines for the scholarly, objective evaluation of nursing research and related literature. This chapter augments Chapter 2 and includes illustrative examples.

Chapter 10
How well do others do it?

APPRAISAL OF RESEARCH REPORTS

Chapter Objectives

Upon successful completion of this chapter the student will be able to

- Critique research done by others with appropriate sensitivity
- Apply principles for critiquing a piece of research
- Use meaningful terms for maximum communication in the critique
- Incorporate a set of guidelines in the critique of nursing research

INTRODUCTION

If the tone of this chapter appears to be much more serious and distant than those that came before, there is a reason: critiquing the work of others is serious. While we can be amusing and flip and have fun with what we do, it is necessary to take on a more objective and scholarly affect as we consider and comment on the works of others.

Two reasons for being quite serious about comments on work done by others are so that we are: (1) not misunderstood; and (2) constructive rather than destructive, instructive rather than obstructive. For example, students respond to comments on papers better if red pencils are not used for making those comments. Ink is even more painful than pencil. Ordinary erasable pencil is less intimidating. Attempts at being funny are not appreciated, and you must have many more positive comments than negative ones for the students to comprehend the positive ones. Also, it's easy to forget to make the positive comments because it is more obvious when something is missing, incorrect, incomprehensible, or confusing. The words "complete," "well-written," "clear," and "comprehensive" are just as easy to write and are sorely needed by the beginning writer.

This chapter will be a discussion of constructive approaches for critiquing nursing research. All research is not good, for any number of reasons. In fact, no research is perfect, particularly nursing research, because nurses study people and people in natural environmemts are impossible to control on even a minimum number of variables. It is important to be able to evaluate studies objectively—not emotionally. Guidelines for the scholarly critique of nursing research will be given. Examples will accompany the guidelines.

CONSTRUCTIVE APPROACHES FOR CRITIQUING NURSING RESEARCH

Two principles to remember when critiquing a piece of research are: be objective, and, make your comments specific to the work you are reviewing. As a nurse, you have been indoctrinated with the importance of objective observations and decisions. The practice is not as easy as it might seem. Suppose you are reviewing an article that is based on a theory that you simply do not "buy." Could you review the article with regard to the research question and the relationship of the question to the conceptual framework (even though you do not agree with the basic premises of the framework)? Could you consider the review of the literature with regard to relevance to the research question and demonstration of the importance of the study?

Could you appraise the research design in terms of appropriateness to the research question? Could you evaluate the presentation of the findings with notation of the appropriateness of the statistical analysis, the adequacy of the discussion, the appropriateness and completeness of the conclusions, and recommendations for further research and practice? Obviously, if you do not agree with the conceptual framework, you might indeed question the study. But could you do so with objectivity?

Leininger (1968) made several pertinent points about the importance of the research critique, the role of the one doing the critique, and the possible reactions of the researcher whose work is critiqued. Leininger defined a research critique as "a critical estimate of a piece of research which has been carefully and systematically studied by a critic who has used specific criteria to appraise the favorable, less favorable, and other general features of the research study" (p. 444). The critique should be objective, of an advisory nature, constructive, and include the strengths, weaknesses, and general features of the research being reviewed. A summary appraisal and recommendations should also be a part of the critique. Understandably, the individual whose work is being critiqued may feel threatened or perceive the critic's comments as explicit recommendations or highly impractical. In spite of the potential emotional reactions to a critique, Leininger believed that "a research critique is an extremely valuable and necessary means to help any researcher develop competence in research as well as for the advancement of a profession" (p. 449).

If, for example, a researcher is investigating the adjustment of postoperative coronary bypass clients to determine how well they are functioning three months after surgery, would crisis theory be an appropriate theoretical framework? Probably not, because most authorities on crisis theory define a crisis as a situation that must be resolved in a relatively short period of time, with six weeks being the outside limit. So right away you might decide that you differ from the thought processes of the researcher. What do you say about the study?

Given that the other elements are adequate, note what those points are and point out that the basic assumptions of crisis theory are not consistent with the focus of the study. If you are scholarly, you will suggest a theoretical framework that will be appropriate. A physiological framework might describe the trauma the heart has experienced, the correction made by the surgery, the healing process including corrections of the disturbances to all body systems and the tissue repair, the optimum exercise and stimulation recommended for the facilitation of the healing process. From this theory, you would make some predictions as to what the desirable and expected level of functioning of such clients would be. With that approach, you will determine how the actual observed functioning, as described by the researcher, matches the theorized functioning and evaluate your theory. Note that this example represents a deductive approach because you began with a theory and collected data to test that theory.

If you are more socially inclined, you could suggest role theory as an appropriate framework for the postoperative coronary bypass clients. Role theory includes the assumption that individuals have parts they play in life. For each role, there is a reciprocal role. For the postoperative client who is home from the hospital, the role he is expected by health care providers to play may be quite different from the role he expects to play and which his family expects him to play. The surgeons and nurses may expect him to eat appropriately, exercise optimally, and maintain an optimistic, cheerful outlook while getting adequate rest and minimizing stress. The client may be concerned about his employment. He may believe that he must immediately have materials brought to him from the office, or indeed, he may insist on going to the office. The energy he spends on the work may prohibit his exercising. The client's family may remember the trauma of this previous heart attack and try to insist that he assume the role of the sick person. These different perceptions of the role expectations of one person from several points of view set up what is known as role conflict. The reviewer might look at the findings and express some hunches as to the role relationships of clients who have shown better functioning behaviors. The same data could possibly be examined from the role theory framework with the outcome of different conclusions and recommendations.

As you critique studies, you will maximize communication if you state that the part is *insufficient* or *inadequate,* meaning it does not cover the material; *illogical,* meaning it does not fit or make sense; *confusing,* meaning it simply is not well expressed; *complex,* meaning it may be more complicated than is necessary, as in trying to combine too many theories or put too much into one design; *inappropriate,* meaning not applicable at that point or not related to the research question or other parts of the study; *invalid,* meaning that the author's interpretation of the data is not in agreement with yours; *questionable,* meaning that there is insufficient data or other evidence for the statements.

Positive terms, in general, are the opposite of the less complimentary ones listed above and have the more favorable connotations. Use the positive terms whenever possible and always say the positive points about a study first. A good way to think about critiquing a study is to discuss the strengths and weaknesses—in that order. Avoid the use of such terms as bad, good, nice, for they do not communicate anything. Statements such as

"The article contained a good review of the literature" do not have any meaning for the reader. (Students often seem very surprised when such noncommunications are criticized by their instructors.) Instead the following brief statement contains much more information: "The researcher included the origin of the word 'empathy,' the various applications that have evolved, and research from three orientations in the review of the literature."

To indicate that the "theoretical framework was appropriate for the research question" is unacceptable. Think how much more informative it is to write: "In order to examine the question of the reasons for the administration of sedatives to hospitalized children by the nurses working night duty, the researcher chose a systems theory framework."

Critiques seem to be difficult to do at first attempts. The reason for the difficulty probably lies in the feeling of insecurity of the beginning critiquer. Well, how do you develop a feeling of competence? Right! You have to practice. Individuals seem to believe that they either can or cannot make scholarly comments. It is unrealistic to expect to be an expert at any skill without practice, and constructive criticism is a skill (Leininger 1968). Remember to be objective and to provide information with your comments. That is, make your comments specific to the work you are reviewing.

To begin the review or critique of a piece of research, think of your task in terms of the purpose of doing it. Are you simply reporting in a general way to a broad audience? Or is your purpose to evaluate the quality of the work in terms of the value of its information to a specific field or topic of interest? In other words, state your case—make an overall statement in relation to your purpose. For example, the reviewer may be pursuing research related to optimal positioning of postlaminectomy clients. The review of an article related to that topic would be from the point of view of the contribution of the article to knowledge about the best position for clients who have undergone a specific type of spinal surgery. The comments might come in the form of the clarity of the recommendations, the tightness of the design, the specificity of the research question, or the relevance to related reviewed research—all with regard to the positioning of postoperative laminectomy clients. In comparison, you could be reviewing the article in order to evaluate the application of a specific theory to nursing practice. In that case, you would examine the relationship of the theory to the design and the findings. Do the findings fit the predictions of the theory? How specifically does theory relate to the findings? Which assumptions of the theory are necessary and which are superfluous? Are any of the assumptions unsupported?

Following the introductory statement, make comments about each part of the research. Note any important elements that are missing and any unnecessary parts that are included.

GUIDELINES FOR A CRITIQUE OF A RESEARCH ARTICLE

[The following set of guidelines has been developed to be a compromise between the extremely detailed guidelines found in such works as Polit and Hungler (1978) and less specific suggestions found elsewhere (Fleming and Hayter 1974), or more aggressive approaches (Strauss 1969).

Definition. A critique is a critical evaluation of a piece of reported research.

Purpose. The purpose of a critique is to communicate the value of the research by identifying and discussing the strengths and weaknesses of each part. In general, the basic parts of a study should be present, clearly and concisely written, and appropriately documented.

Outline. The basic parts of a critique are

1. *Problem.* Identify the problem and discuss the problem statement in terms of clarity, appropriateness, and relevance to nursing.

2. *Purpose.* What is the specified purpose and its relationship to the problem statement? Is this purpose appropriate for investigation?

3. *Conceptual framework.* What is the conceptual framework? How does it relate to the problem?

4. *Review of the literature.* What are the primary sources reviewed? How do they relate to the problem? Are previous studies adequately critiqued? What does the study being critiqued add to what is already in the literature?

5. *Hypothesis.* What is (are) the hypothesis (ses) and/or research question(s)? What is the rationale for this selection?

6. *Variables.* Identify the independent and dependent variables. Note the controlled and confounding variables as identified in the study or as implied but not discussed. Define the important variables. Are uncontrolled variables identified?

7. *Methodology*

   a) What kind of design is used? Discuss its appropriateness according to the variables studied and the purpose of the investigation.

b) How were the variables measured? What instruments were used? Discuss the validity and reliability of the instruments.

c) What was the population of this study? How was the sample drawn? Discuss the appropriateness of the sample as representative of the population.

d) What was the procedure of collecting the data? What additional information (if any) would you need in order to replicate the study?

e) How were the rights, comfort, and convenience of the subjects assured?

8. *Findings*

a) Describe the subjects including number and demographic information.

b) What were the data collected? How were the data analyzed? How did the analysis of the data relate to the research hypothesis (ses) and/or question(s)?

c) How did the researcher interpret the findings? Was the interpretation appropriate (i.e., based on the data)? Are there other plausible explanations for the findings?

d) What were the conclusions drawn by the researcher?

9. *Discussion.* Note how the researcher related the findings to the problem and the purpose of the study. How did the researcher relate the findings to the literature review? Were there any unexpected findings that were outside the original purpose of the study? If so, what were these serendipitous findings?

10. *Recommendations.* What were the suggestions made by the researcher for nursing practice and for further research? Were these suggestions appropriately based on the findings of this study?

11. *Summary.* Make some concluding evaluation statement as to the overall worth and relevance of the study.

Note also that many authorities are suggesting that the qualifications of the researcher be included in the critique. However desirable that suggestion may be, it is often impossible to infer or question expertise based on the limited information usually provided in journals.

SUMMARY

With the research process ready to recycle with the critique phase, a very important concept pervades the process and will be discussed in Part IV. Chapter 11 provides rationale and guidelines for ethical considerations in nursing research.

Suggestions for Further Study

1. Critique the reports of your peers and have them critique your report. Were their suggestions helpful? Were there some comments with which you disagreed? How did you feel during the process of the criticism?

2. Have a small group discussion critiquing an article from a recent nursing research journal. Decide on the article prior to the discussion and give everyone a chance to read it.

3. Think critically about everything you read and hear.

Suggestions for Additional Readings

Brink, P. J., and Wood, M. J. *Basic Steps in Planning Nursing Research from Question to Proposal* (2nd edition). Monterey, CA: Wadsworth Health Sciences Division, 1983. (Chapter 4)

Fleming, J. W., and Hayter, J. "Reading Research Reports Critically," *Nursing Outlook,* 1974, *22*(3), pp. 172–175.

Fox, D. J. *Fundamentals of Research in Nursing* (4th edition). Norwalk, CN: Appleton-Century-Crofts, 1982. (Chapter 7)

Komnenich, P., and Noack, J. A. "The Process of Critiquing," in S. D. Krampitz and N. Pavlovich (Eds.), *Readings for Nursing Research.* St. Louis: The C. V. Mosby Company, 1981.

Leininger, M. M. "The Research Critique: Nature, Function, and Art," *Nursing Research,* 1968, *17*(5), pp. 444–449.

Mallick, M. J. "A Constant Comparative Method for Teaching Research Critique to Baccalaureate Nursing Students," *Image,* 1983, *15*(4), pp. 120–123.

Polit, D. F., and Hungler, B. P. *Nursing Research: Principles and Methods* (2nd edition). Philadelphia: J. B. Lippincott Company, 1983. (Chapter 26)

Strauss, S. "Guidelines for Analysis of Research Reports," *The Journal of Educational Research,* 1969, *63*(4), pp. 165–169.

PART IV
ETHICAL CONSIDERATIONS OF NURSING RESEARCH

Nurses are faced with more ethical dilemmas now than in the past. The number is expected to increase as nurses assume more autonomy and as health science makes possible the prolongation of life with the quality of life sometimes questionable. This fourth part of the book is designed to acquaint the nurse researcher with ethical considerations inherent in conducting research.

The first consideration is that the nurse has a responsibility to provide the best care possible for clients. In order to determine what care is best, the nurse must be aware of advances made by others in providing care, must be able to evaluate those advances, and must do some investigations in areas where others have not delved. Implicit in the latter responsibility is the admonition to be as well qualified as possible and to know one's strengths and limitations. With such knowledge one will know when and where to seek advice and information as indicated—from the research facilitator, the statistician, the clinician, or the expert in some other discipline.

When the nurse conducts the research, there is the responsibility to design the study as effectively and efficiently as possible in order to

- minimize inconvenience, discomfort, and time imposed on clients (subjects)
- maximize findings
- maximize relevance of findings to theory, the works of others, and nursing practice

Nurses are *the best* qualified professionals to conduct research into a number of areas. These primary nursing research fields include

- health promotion and care of elderly individuals
- physical and mental health promotion and care of severely mentally handicapped adults and children
- health promotion of mentally retarded children and adults
- promotion of adaptive coping behaviors by physically handicapped individuals
- mental and physical health promotion and care of individuals with chronic and degenerative illnesses

Chapter 11 contains an introduction to the principles of ethics as applicable to nursing research. An example of ethical dilemmas faced by one nurse researcher are included to illustrate the problems and the application of the principles.

Chapter 11
Can you do research while continuing to be a kind, caring nurse?

CONSIDERATION OF OTHERS—KEEPING IT ALL IN PERSPECTIVE

Chapter Objectives

Upon successful completion of this chapter the student will be able to

- Discuss the potential role conflict for the nurse as the researcher *and* the patient's advocate
- Relate ethical considerations to federal guidelines for conducting research on human subjects
- Discuss the elements of informed consent
- List the levels of moral justification
- Define and apply four moral principles

INTRODUCTION

Throughout this text, we have attempted to emphasize the responsibility of the nurse to do research. There are other considerations that will be addressed in this chapter. Specifically, the nurse must maintain a delicate balance between the rights of the individual and the potential benefits findings may have for society. The problem has been expressed that, as nurses, it is hard to be in the research role while at the same time we are in the patient-advocate role.

Suppose, for example, that you are a nurse researcher observing the behaviors of nurses as they care for dying patients. You are not providing any care, a fact that has been made clear to the clients and the nurses. In order for you to make your observations, you must be in the client's room while the nurse is providing care. All of the indicated consent forms have been signed by the appropriate individuals. You observe the nurse who is responsible for the client as that nurse violates principles of aseptic care in the irrigation of a Foley catheter. What is your ethical responsibility as a researcher? As a nurse? To the client?

If you are a person who wants *the* answer, ethical considerations (and research per se) will be very frustrating for you. If you are an individual who really gets excited about a philosophical issue and enjoys a lively debate, ethical dilemmas are for you. A dilemma is by definition "a situation involving choice between equally unsatisfactory alternatives" (*Webster's New Collegiate Dictionary* 1961, p. 232). There are principles to guide decisions that will make the choices somewhat more defensible.

FEDERAL GUIDELINES

While the emphasis on ethical considerations has increased since 1976 when the United States Department of Health, Education and Welfare (HEW, now known as the Department of Health and Human Services or HHS) issued a set of regulations for the protection of human subjects in research, ethical dilemmas are not new. Fox (1982) identifies Eve's eating the forbidden fruit as the first recorded example of an ethical dilemma. Fox continues with an exceptionally inclusive historical treatment of the development of ethical guidelines for research.

The HEW guidelines indicated that research would not be considered acceptable unless the benefits outweighed the risks involved. Subsequently these initial guidelines have been expanded to include special considerations for compensation of injured research subjects (1977), research on the fetus (1976), research involving prisoners (1976), psychosurgery (1977), research involving children (1977), and research involving those institutionalized as mentally infirm (1978). Institutional review boards were established in each institution receiving federal funding for research. Among the provisions of these regulations was the requirement of obtaining *informed consent* from each subject. Potential subjects must be informed of the potential risks involved in the participation in the research, and they must be apprised of benefits they might gain from participation or the lack of benefits to subjects. Obtaining consent implies the rights of the potential subjects to refuse to participate without penalty or censure.

INFORMED CONSENT

If obtaining informed consent seems easy, you are deceived. To complicate and make a point of the seriousness of the process, the elements of informed consent as identified by Beauchamp and Childress (1979) are presented and discussed. The *information elements* are (1) disclosure of information and (2) comprehension of information. The *consent elements* are (1) voluntary consent and (2) competence to consent. Think about the element of disclosure of information. If you tell subjects exactly what the study is about, what the hypotheses are, are you not biasing the study? How do you resolve the problem of informed consent while maintaining the integrity of your design?

The subjects should be informed of the *purpose* of the study. The wording of the purpose becomes important. The purpose may be stated in terms such as "to gather information to improve the care of clients in the intensive care unit." In this example, the researcher may be concerned with the quality of care in the intensive care unit, but it is not necessary to put the purpose in negative terms for the client. It is necessary to avoid deception. You may *not* tell the nurses that you are there to observe client behavior when, in fact, you are there to observe the nurses as they provide care. The clients must be informed as to what they are expected to do if they participate in the study. Will there be procedures for them to undergo? Drugs to take? A questionnaire to complete (if so, how long is the questionnaire and how long does it usually take to complete)? Will there be interviews? By whom? How long will the interview take? What are the nature of the interview questions? If the questions are sensitive, the potential subject must be informed of that fact before being asked to grant consent. In summary, informed means that the potential subject is presented in writing with a non-deceptive explanation of the purpose of the study and what the researcher is requesting that the subject undergo or do, with the time involvement specified and the risks and benefits (or absence thereof) clearly indicated.

The second information element, comprehension of information, is difficult to measure. In fact, there is reason to believe that clients frequently sign consent forms that clearly specify the procedures that the client is agreeing to, but they have no understanding of the nature of the operation they are agreeing to undergo. The explanation must be in terms the potential subject understands. If the subject is not fluent in English (or whatever language you are using), the explanation must be translated into the subject's primary language or one in which the subject is fluent. Professional jargon must be omitted or defined in terms the subject understands. (Explaining things in understandable language is something at which nurses, in comparison to other health professionals, often excel.) Potential subjects with less education than average must have the explanation at their level. The information must be read to potential subjects who cannot read for any reason—eyesight impairment or lack of reading comprehension skills.

Children must be informed and consent obtained in an appropriate way, depending on the child's developmental level. Children who can sign a consent form should be requested to do so. Any child should be informed of exactly what is going to happen to him or her and what he or she is expected to do. For children who cannot sign a consent form, verbal consent must be obtained. Permission must also be obtained from the parent or guardian of a minor. Such permission is also part of the consent procedure, and a space on the subject consent form should be available for the signature of the parent or guardian. This consent is mandatory and, in practice, not usually difficult to obtain.

The *voluntary consent element* presupposes that the potential subjects are truly acting freely, that is, free of any coercion or threat thereof. Individuals must believe that if they refuse to participate in the study, no censure will be imposed. Clients in a hospital or other institution are extremely vulnerable. They have, in a sense, placed themselves into the hands of others (or been placed there). Often persons believe that they must consent to anything suggested in order to be considered a "good" client and receive the rewards of being good—meals, medications, privileges, or information. Not only must the researcher assure the individuals that no censure will be imposed, but that in fact must be true. In your enthusiasm for your project, you must not lose sight of the rights of others, but must always show respect for their dignity.

Students are frequently asked to participate in a study, particularly students in a research course. Are they free to refuse? What happens to those who do not choose to participate? The only safe way to safeguard the students' autonomy is by designing the procedure so that the instructor/researcher does not know who participates and who does not. This problem can be addressed by passing out the subject consent forms with the questionnaire and instructions for the students to detach the consent forms from the questionnaire and place them in separate boxes in "neutral" locations. Neutral means somewhere other than the instructor/researcher's office or the classroom during class. The faculty mailbox is safe because it is away from the faculty offices and students could place the materials in the faculty boxes without revealing participation or lack thereof. The obvious flaw with this system is that an instructor could conceivably go through the consent forms to determine who did not sign one. The same problem occurs in the hospital where the researcher as well as staff will know who participates in a study and who does not. Researchers simply must be scrupulously honest and careful to preserve autonomy and anonymity of subjects and potential subjects.

The *competence to consent* element is an even more complex concept. Recognizing the ambiguity of the term and the difficulty in applying the concept of competence in diverse situations, Beauchamp and Childress (1979) suggested the following guideline:

> A person is competent if and only if that person can make decisions based on rational reasons. In biomedical contexts this standard entails that a person must be able to understand a therapy or research procedure, must be able to weigh its risks and benefits, and must be able to make a decision in the light of such knowledge and through such abilities, even if the person chooses not to utilize the information. (p. 69)

This standard is helpful, but how does one determine if a person is able to understand? Can clients with organic brain syndrome, mental illness, development disabilities, sensory deficits "understand" a therapy much less be able to weigh risks and benefits and make a decision based on rational reasons?

The problem occurs frequently in clinical research. Researchers studying attitudes of residents of homes for elderly citizens find that many of these individuals have legal guardians, who may be children or others who live some distance away and visit infrequently. It would seem to be important to obtain consent from such guardians just as one would obtain consent from the guardian or parent of a ten-year-old child; however, these elderly individuals are not children and are often competent according to the standard of being able to make a decision based on rational reasons. Sometimes the agency or someone within the agency is the legal guardian. Since the agency presumably has granted you permission to conduct the study, it may be simpler to obtain guardian consent in such cases. Whoever or whatever the legal guardian, it is necessary to obtain consent from the individuals themselves at whatever level they are capable of responding. Some will be quite capable of signing a consent form, and some will need to have the form read to them; others will want to discuss it, and there will be those who will simply nod assent.

LEVELS OF MORAL JUSTIFICATION

Beauchamp and Childress (1979) have developed what they termed levels of moral justification. These are (1) judgments and actions; (2) rules; (3) principles; (4) ethical theories. "According to this diagram, judgments about what ought to be done in particular situations are justified by moral rules, which in turn are grounded in principles and ultimately in ethical theories" (p. 5).

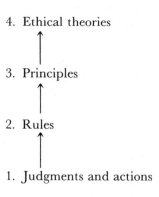

4. Ethical theories

3. Principles

2. Rules

1. Judgments and actions

A *judgment* is a decision, verdict, or conclusion about a particular action. *Rules* state that actions of a certain kind ought (or ought not) to be done because they are right (or wrong). *Principles* are more general and fundamental than moral rules and serve as the foundation for the rules. *Theories* are bodies of principles and rules, more or less systematically related (p. 5). Consider the example given by Beauchamp and Childress.

> A physician who refuses to perform amniocentesis (*judgment* and resulting refusal to perform a given *action*) may maintain that it is morally wrong intentionally to kill innocent human beings. When pressed, he may justify the proclaimed moral *rule* against killing innocent human beings by reference to a *principle* of the sanctity of

human life. Finally, the particular *judgment,* the *rule,* and the *principle* may be grounded in an *ethical theory.* (p. 5—paraphrased)

In considering these levels of moral justification in more depth, let's start with the broad base; that is, the theories. Two moral theories that serve as the basis for many judgments and actions are the theories of utilitarianism and deontology. Beauchamp and Childress (1979) use the term "utilitarianism" to refer

> to the moral theory that there is one and only one basic principle in ethics, the principle of utility. This principle asserts that we ought in all circumstances to produce the greatest possible balance of value over disvalue for all persons affected (or the least possible balance of disvalue if only evil results can be brought about). (p. 21)

As Beauchamp and Childress (1979) indicate, there is disagreement among utilitarians concerning how this theory may be characterized best, as well as disputes over which values are most important. In short, the theory is complicated because of several differing schools of utilitarians. Application is not always consistent, but the emphasis appears to be on the outcome or the consequences.

In contrast, deontological theories maintain that at least some acts are wrong and others are right independent of their consequences. Examples given by Beauchamp and Childress (1979) of right-making characteristics in deontological systems include fidelity to promises and contracts, gratitude for benefits received, truthfulness, and justice. All of those examples sound like traits most of us could applaud, but think about it. If you follow the deontological theory and never engage in any deceit, you could never give a client a placebo. You could never encourage a client whose condition you believed to be hopeless. In research, the placebo problem is dealt with by telling all subjects that some will be getting the placebo and others will be getting the experimental drug so that no one is deceived about the design of the study. After the study, it is important to have a debriefing to inform all of the subjects about the findings and offer the experimental drug to those who received the placebo, if in fact the findings were interpreted as indicating that the experimental drug had a safe and favorable effect. Be aware that this definition and example of deontological theory is greatly simplified. For a more thorough discussion, Beauchamp and Childress' 1979 book is recommended.

The next level of moral justification is that of *principles.* Beauchamp and Childress (1979) list the following moral principles and definitions thereof:

1. The *principle of autonomy* includes the aspect of the individual's self-regarding actions which ought to be as free as possible so that one can do as one wishes. The aspect of evaluation of the self-regarding actions of others is such that we ought to respect them as persons with the same right to their judgments as we have to our own.

2. The *principle of nonmaleficence* is associated with the maxim "above all, do not harm" and includes the admonition to be thoughtful and act carefully.

3. The *principle of beneficence* is used to refer to acts involving prevention of harm, removal of harmful conditions, and positive benefiting.

4. The *principle of justice* is that everyone should get what is deserved or one's "just dessert."

There are other moral principles that are relevant to the health care provider. The principles presented are much more complex than the definitions might indicate. For example, how do you decide what one's just dessert is? Do you distribute goods on the basis of need, merit, equality, or social contribution? What are the criteria for establishing whichever basis you choose? For example, if you choose to distribute goods on the basis of need, what are the criteria for determining need?

In research these principles should be of concern and applicable at a very basic level. Above all, do no harm and whenever possible do good. Respect each individual as a person and make the opportunities to participate in research, as well as the benefits of research, available to those who deserve it.

REALITIES THAT COMPLICATE ETHICAL DILEMMAS IN NURSING RESEARCH

The moral principles seem basic. It would appear that there should never be a question of any nurse following these basic principles of biomedical ethics. Nevertheless, there are pressures on the nurse researcher that could cause nurses to lose sight of the basic goal of health promotion. Dr. Elizabeth Sharp (class presentation 1982) identified the following pressures that must be recognized and dealt with in order for the nurse researcher to keep research efforts in the proper perspective.

1. The pressure to publish is growing and competition to get an article in a refereed journal is becoming increasingly difficult.

2. In order to publish, there is the pressure to produce meaningful data—hence the threat of fraud. Remember that you are responsible for the data you present even if you have had someone else collect the data for you. It is important to have only well-qualified and trustworthy assistants working with you.

3. During the process of data collection, you may want to change your criteria for the admission of individuals to your study because of difficulty in getting the number of subjects desired who meet your criteria. You may also wish to decrease the number of subjects you have originally planned to include. Either change is a change in your design and is a serious decision. The decision must be based on some of the principles of moral research conduct. For example, if you decide to stop data collection after collection from 14 subjects instead of the 25 you had planned to include there are several ramifications you must consider: (a) permission to conduct the study from each research committee you passed through is based on the number of subjects you originally projected, to do less is a breach of contract; (b) the findings are not as likely to show significant results with fewer subjects which means that the time and efforts of the subjects who did participate is not as well used as it would be if you continued your study and had a more significant and generalizable set of data. There are no easy answers; contracts can be renegotiated and trade-offs are sometimes necessary in order to get results analyzed within some meaningful time frame. The point is that you are changing your contract and commitment when you change your design so do not make any changes without due consideration and without adequate negotiations with all of the involved committees and agency representatives.

AN EXAMPLE OF ETHICAL ISSUES INVOLVED IN NURSING RESEARCH

A study involving the informed consent of mothers of newborn baby boys provided multiple ethical decisions. The researcher, Brenda Knaack (1982), questioned whether mothers who signed consent forms to have their infant sons circumcised were truly *informed;* that is, did they fully understand the benefits and the risks involved. The benefits are questioned because of the statement by the American Academy of Pediatrics that there is no apparent benefit to circumcision. The procedure is not without risks. Knaack based her study on the assumption that society is not properly informed about the benefits and risks of circumcision and the implication that society has the right to be informed. What is good for society might not be beneficial to the institution (in this case the hospital whose staff assumed that baby boys would be circumcised except for religious reasons). The design was experimental, with an experimental and a control group. Both groups completed a pretest. The experimental group was subsequently given information about circumcision (that is, they were *informed*), while the control group was given no additional information other than what the staff routinely told the mothers in order to obtain consent signatures. The dependent variable was the number of mothers who consented or refused consent for their sons to be circumcised. The design had internal validity problems because it is not clear whether the administration of the pretest itself might change the views and thence the decision to have the baby circumcised. Another ethical consideration was the incorrect answers the control group might give on the multiple choice examination. Would choosing an incorrect answer strengthen the beliefs of the subjects in that incorrect position?

An unexpected situation arose as Knaack discovered that the subjects did not know what circumcision was. Some of the definitions they gave were bizarre. What is the researcher's ethical responsibility in such circumstances? Another problem arose in adhering to the study criteria, since to stick to the established criteria would eliminate subjects with certain characteristics. An unanticipated situation arose as evidence of stress and frustration of the subjects was observed. As the subjects became informed, they questioned the need for circumcision. However, their families, including the fathers of the babies, put much pressure on the mothers to conform to society's expectation of having the babies circumcised.

Because of these ethical dilemmas, Knaack decided to stop the study short of the original number of subjects planned. It appeared that the stress on the subjects was too great to warrant continuation of the research.

Knaack's experiences serve as an example of how ethical decisions impact on a problem identified for investigation. The problem was a researchable one, the design well-planned, but the frustration experienced by the subjects was not anticipated. The resistance of the hospital staff to the challenges in the routine was expected, but the decision to do the study was based on what was believed to be in the best interest of society. The principle of above all do no harm (nonmalevolence) was invoked in the decision to curtail the frustrations of any other subjects.

SUMMARY

Grappling with the issues related to ethics requires abstract thinking and ability to debate principles in situations where answers are not easy. For nurses who are ready for a challenge, this area is open and is surely challenging.

Just before you leave the idea of nursing research and become a nurse ethicist, read Chapter 12 and reconsider nursing research. The areas are not mutually exclusive—you could do both.

Suggestions for Further Study

Ethical dilemmas are excellent topics for discussion because there are no obvious answers and because new angles will emerge in each new discussion. Consider the following situations and discuss with peers how you would make a decision and what principles you would be basing that decision on.

1. Go back to the situation posed at the beginning of this chapter and, after discussion, decide what you would do and what principles you would be applying. You need not be confined to the principles listed in this book; think of some that you use such as "one should always tell the truth."

2. In the chapter the reasons for not decreasing the number of subjects originally projected were presented. Yet, in the example given of Knaack's (1982) study, the decision was made to curtail the study. Discuss the principles involved. Do you agree with Knaack's decision? Why or why not?

Suggestions for Additional Reading

Beauchamp, T. L., and Childress, J. F. *Principles of Biomedical Ethics.* New York: Oxford University Press, 1979.

Fox, D. J. *Fundamentals of Research in Nursing* (4th edition). Norwalk, CN: Appleton-Century-Crofts, 1982. (Chapter 4)

Treece, E. W., and Treece, J. W. *Elements of Research in Nursing.* St. Louis: The C. V. Mosby Company, 1982.

PART V
APPLICATION OF RESEARCH FINDINGS TO CLINICAL PRACTICE

The fifth part of this book is designed to stimulate the nurse to make intelligent applications of research findings in clinical practice. No matter how much fun research may be, it is all for naught if the findings are not applied as indicated. Resistance to change is well documented and makes the application of findings difficult. The lack of application results in duplication of effort, continuance in antiquated methods of care, and delayed progress in the growth of the science of nursing.

Chapter 12 contains an elaboration of the cautions and responsibilities associated with the application of research findings. As the last chapter in the book, it completes the research cycle by referring back to the first chapter. The concept that most clearly ties in with Chapter 1 is the idea of the generation of research ideas in the clinical practice area. The application of research findings in nursing practice will inevitably generate new questions that will stimulate nurses to seek answers through the research process.

Chapter 12
Why go through all this anyway?

NECESSITY OF NURSING RESEARCH

Chapter Objectives

Upon successful completion of this chapter the student will be able to

- Give reasons why nursing research is important
- Identify the various ways nurses can be involved in research so that *any* nurse who wishes can participate
- Give an example of some meaningful research being done
- Anticipate and prepare for the resistances nurses will meet as they try to do research

INTRODUCTION

When the original outline of this text was shared with a nursing leader, it only contained the first 11 chapters. This person suggested that with all of the "what's" a "why" was indicated. That's true, but the "why" is more difficult to write. There are few doubts about the research process (although the sequence and emphasis varies considerably), but the why of nursing research is much more personal and must be answered by each of us.

IMPORTANCE OF NURSING RESEARCH

As indicated in Chapter 1, improved client care is the "bottom line" of all we do. All other activity is peripheral. The primary importance of nursing research is just that—to improve client care. In addition, the reduction of health care costs is of grave concern, as costs are escalating so rapidly. Although other professionals could and do conduct research to improve client care and reduce costs, only nurses doing research will contribute to the development of the nursing profession.

Improved Health Care and Reduced Cost

One obvious reason for nursing research is for the good of *society*. Nurses must ask questions about their practices and seek systematic answers in order to improve nursing care and promote health. Society has demonstrated little awareness of the responsibility nurses have for the critical decisions that must be made on the spot in critical care units. Highly skilled nurses are the ones who make the difference in the recovery rates of postoperative clients. We need research to show these facts. Nurses are the professionals who are concerned with the maternal and paternal infant bonding that must occur for healthy family relationships. Yes, other professionals have done studies related to the subject, but nurses are with mothers during delivery and with the newborns in the nurseries and are the ones who are in the best positions to facilitate the bonding. There is a need to produce more studies to convince the public that nursing makes a difference.

Claire Fagin has collected nursing studies that demonstrate the economic value of nursing research. A colleague described Fagin's presentation of her project at the Council of Nurse Researchers meeting at the Biennial Convention of the American Nurses' Association in 1982 as giving "pride and inspiration like nothing else I know of. It also is wonderful information for MD's and the laity who wonder what nurses can possibly do research on." The overwhelming evidence presented by Fagin was that nurses are economical as staff, nursing interventions can save enormous amounts of money, and investment in nursing research pays impressive dividends.

Fagin's review of studies evaluating primary nursing care revealed remarkably consistent results. One study reported was assessment of primary nursing on the postoperative adaptation of renal transplant patients. The subjects, who were cared for in a primary nursing arrangement, went home a full three weeks before the subjects who received traditional, routinely organized care. In addition, the group receiving traditional care had a mean of 4.6 complications after surgery, while the group receiving primary nursing care had a mean of 1.4 complications after surgery. The actual expense figures for one year for the very small group of patients involved in this study revealed a financial savings of $51,084.80. Another study in a hospital in a Chicago suburb, changed from an 82 percent RN staff to a 100 percent RN staff. A cost savings of $83,788.00 over a four-year period was identified for one unit studied. Other organizational benefits resulting from the change to an all-RN staff included reduction in total numbers of personnel required to staff the units, reduced turnover, and increased credentials of RN staff. Although some details are missing, the dollar savings are impressive. In fact, all the research reviewed showed the significant economic value of both primary nursing and an all-, or higher ratio of, RN staff.

The potential savings in health care of interventions designed and tested by nurses is even more impressive. Is 52 millions of dollars a year meaningful? One nursing intervention can save that much! In association with colleagues, Gene Cranston Anderson of the University of Florida did a series of studies on the effects of nonnutritive sucking of premature infants. In one study (Measel and Anderson 1979) 30 infants were allowed to suck on a pacifier before and after each tube feeding. They were compared with a control group who received routine care which included few, if any, sucking opportunities. The experimental group infants were home eight days sooner than those in the control group, at an actual cost savings of $3,494 each, or $104,000 total. Since at least 15,000 infants similar to these are born in the United States each year, the potential cost savings is $52 million!

The work of Ida Martinson (1978) in the home care of dying children has been impressive for some time. In addition to being so humane, so caring, and so nursing, home care, her work has shown, also saves money. Hospital care was 18 times more expensive than home care. For the children studied, the actual mean cost was $13,022 per child for hospital care, as compared to a mean cost of $827 for each child who died at home. As Fagin pointed out, "the cost benefits are superseded by the human value" in studies such as Martinson's.

Fagin has made a great case for nursing research being cost effective. Considering the hospital cash flow, the amount of money that could be saved by even one study (e.g., Measel and Anderson 1979) justifies the moneys invested in nursing research. Considering the financial support of nursing research from the point of view of how much of the hospital budget goes for such projects, the facts are appalling. No major industry has invested so little in research that is so central to its primary purpose.

To understand more fully how nursing can be used in nursing practice, consider the Conduct and Utilization of Research in Nursing (CURN) Project from Michigan (Horsley, Crane, and Haller 1981–1982). Working with 32 nursing departments in hospitals throughout the state, the use of research to improve nursing practice was tested. Ten research-based protocols were developed and tested.

1. Structured preoperative teaching
2. A lactose-free diet
3. Sensation information: distress reduction
4. Sensory information: recovery rate
5. Nonsterile intermittent urinary catheterization
6. Prevention of catheter-associated urinary tract infections
7. Intravenous cannula change regimen
8. Prevention of decubiti by means of small shifts of body weight
9. Mutual goal setting: goal attainment
10. Deliberative nursing: pain reduction

A monograph has been prepared for each of these areas.

Development of Professional Nursing

The next group to whom we must address the importance of nursing research is the *profession*. We need to increase the body of nursing knowledge (surely you have heard this issue addressed previously). Is nursing a science? If so, why? If not, why not? Those are questions that have been and are being debated. Whatever the answer, research is needed to enhance the recognition of nursing as a science. Such recognition would increase respectability and draw the brightest, most motivated, and best qualified students from the resource pools. These students would do outstanding research, which would impress legislators, who would appropriate more funding for nursing research; nurses would, thus, be known as scholars and scientists. The possibilities are unlimited.

Closely related to the opportunities for the profession are the positions of schools of nursing on university campuses. Several well known and respected schools of nursing have closed due to the economic factors of decreased funding from the federal government which has threatened the very existence of some private universities. Schools of nursing are considered to be costly. Research in these schools would serve to increase their status, and society tends to be willing to pay for high-status institutions. Research into innovative educational methods could decrease the cost of nursing schools and thus preserve the schools within university settings. Research is expected of university faculty members, and nursing cannot plead to be an exception. Nursing faculty must produce research in order to attain and maintain the full rights and privileges of university faculty.

The new phenomenon of prospective-payment system, known as the diagnostic related group (DRG) system, is having an impact on nursing. Nursing services consume up to 30 percent of hospital budgets, making nursing a significant item when cost containment is at issue. In addition to the panic the DRGs are creating in some nurses, the potential (no, the imperative) for research is obvious. Documentation of what nurses do for patients with what health problem is necessary. What about the relationship of the DRGs to the studies cited by Fagin in which staffing patterns with all-, or high ratio of, RN staff resulted in cost saving? What are the implications for staffing patterns? What will tighter controls do to morale, turnover, client satisfaction, and rate of recovery? The potential for research is unlimited!

There is the negative implication for research under the DRG system. If nurses have to be so conscious of spending all their time on nursing functions, is research going to have a high enough priority to justify nurses' time and effort?

INVOLVEMENT OF NURSES IN RESEARCH

Clinical settings where research is produced are better known and considered more prestigious than those having nothing to show to the world. Nurses must be involved in the research produced. There are several levels of potential involvement for nurses: (1) as subjects who are demonstrating different approaches of nursing care; (2) as data collectors for research being conducted by others; (3) as research collaborators with individuals from other disciplines such as medicine, pharmacology, social work, psychology, or physical therapy (There are examples of research done by nurses and members of each of these disciplines.); and (4) as the initiators and directors of research.

Career ladders and other schemes to retain nurses and enrich jobs often have research involvement built into the rungs. There has been great increase in hospitals hiring directors of nursing research or starting joint appointments in research with faculty from nursing schools.

At Massachusetts General Hospital, a Nursing Studies Program has been organized to facilitate the involvement of nurses in research (Stetler 1984). Various strategies have been tested since 1980. Continuing education programs have been developed and innovative methods of helping nurses use research has been successful. This program includes "outside" research—from students outside the hospital and research initiated by hospital nursing staff. The nursing staff who have participated in the project have expressed a greater understanding of the importance of nursing research and an increased ability to critique nursing research.

All of the levels of reasons for nursing research are important. But perhaps the one that has the most appeal is the desire to seek answers to questions, to discover new truths, to identify new relationships, to create, and to learn. This appeal on the individual level is where nursing research must begin for each nurse. Only if individuals become curious and motivated will the needed nursing research be conducted. Some individuals will be influential because of their interest in and support of others who are doing the research. Supporters are necessary and their role should be recognized and applauded.

IT'S NOT GOING TO BE EASY

You need to know before you go out to revolutionize health care and nursing practice that it is not going to be easy. The reason for including this word of warning is so that you will not be discouraged. Guess where your greatest opposition will come. Right! From other nurses. It is hard to know why; or rather, to consider all of the possible reasons here. Nevertheless, it is true that nurses will resist change, they will criticize the nurse who is studying the "obvious." Nurses will say that if the research nurses would spend more time caring for the clients instead of sitting in the library or "just observing," it would make the work easier for those who are working. Someone will say "Can you believe the government (or a foundation or the agency) is *paying* for those nurses to play with numbers or punch a calculator!" It's okay. You are used to being questioned about your behavior. Your father wanted to know why you wanted to be a nurse in the first place, and your friends cannot understand why you are having to work so much harder to get a degree in nursing than they are working to achieve a high grade point average in liberal arts. Just explain that it is important to document the tremendous contributions nurses and nursing are making to promote health, relieve suffering, and provide a healing environment. Realize that they cannot understand, avoid being defensive, and do what is right for you.

SUMMARY

This chapter is not intended to be the last—it is meant to be a beginning of research consumption and production by you. You will need much more information, experience, and advice, but you have made a beginning. The more involved you become in research, the more you will realize there is to be done.

Suggestions for Further Study

This is the end of this book. Hopefully, there will be parts to which you will refer until you move on to a more advanced level; so do not throw the book away, yet. The best suggestion for further study is to push you to go do nursing research. The other research books referenced throughout this volume will serve as helpful resources. In addition, you will want to seek advice from clinical experts, researchers, and statisticians, and probably many others as indicated.

Identify at least one nurse researcher whose work interests you. Talk with that person, or write if talking is not possible. Find out how you can do a similar study, participate in the research of that investigator, or develop some related idea. Most nurse researchers are eager to discuss their works with anyone who is interested; if you should happen to approach one who is not encouraging, find someone else. Do not be discouraged if you find you get more questions than answers from "the experts." Raising questions is what research is all about.

Suggestions for Additional Reading

Fawcett, J. "Utilization of Nursing Research Findings," *Image,* 1982, *14*(2), pp. 57–59.

Gaynor, J. M., Kant, D. A., and Mills, E. M. "DRGs: Regulatory and Budgetary Adjustments," *Nursing and Health Care,* 1984, *5*(5), pp. 275–279.

Hamilton, J. M. "Nursing and DRGs: Proactive Responses to Prospective Reimbursement," *Nursing and Health Care,* 1984, *5*(3), pp. 155–159.

Horsley, J. A., Crane, J., and Haller, K. B. *Conduct and Utilization of Research in Nursing Project.* New York: Grune & Stratton, 1981.

Martinson, I. M., Armstrong, G. D., Geis, D. P., Anglin, M. A., Grouseth, E. C., MacInnis, H., Nesbit, M. E., and Kersey, J. H. "Facilitating Home Care for Children Dying of Cancer," *Cancer Nursing,* 1978, *1,* pp. 41–45.

Measel, C. P., and Anderson, G. C. "Nonnutritive Sucking during Tube Feedings: Effect upon Clinical Course in Premature Infants," *Journal of Obstetric, Gynecologic and Neonatal Nursing,* 1979, *8,* pp. 265–272.

Stetler, C. B. *Nursing Research in a Service Setting.* Reston, VA: Reston Publishing Company, Inc., 1984.

Toth, R. M. "DRGs: Imperative Strategies for Nursing Service Administration," *Nursing and Health Care,* 1984, *5*(4), pp. 197–203.

REFERENCES

Abbott, N. K. "Findings, Conclusions, and Recommendations," in S. D. Krampitz and N. Pavlovich (Eds.), *Readings for Nursing Research.* St. Louis: The C. V. Mosby Company, 1981.

Abdellah, F. G., and Levine, E. *Better Patient Care through Nursing Research* (2nd edition). New York: The Macmillan Company, 1979.

Beauchamp, T. L., and Childress, J. F. *Principles of Biomedical Ethics.* New York: Oxford University Press, 1979.

Bertalanffy, L. "General Systems Theory: A Critical Review," in W. Buckley (Ed.), *Modern Systems Research for the Behavioral Scientist.* Chicago: Aldine, 1968.

Binger, J. L., and Jensen, L. M. *Lippincott's Guide to Nursing Literature.* Philadelphia: J. B. Lippincott Company, 1980.

Brink, P. J., and Wood, M. J. *Basic Steps in Planning Nursing Research from Question to Proposal* (2nd edition). Monterey, CA: Wadsworth Health Sciences Division, 1983.

Brogan, D. "Choosing an Appropriate Statistical Test of Significance for a Nursing Research Hypothesis or Question," *Western Journal of Nursing Research,* 1981, *3*(4), pp. 337–369.

Buros, O. (Ed.). *The Eighth Mental Measurement Yearbook.* Hyland Park, NJ: Gryphon Press, 1978.

Butts, P. A. "Dissemination of Nursing Research Findings, *Image,* 1982, *14*(2), pp. 62–64.

deLemos, H. F. *Effectiveness of Human Sexuality Training Workshops Led by a Nurse for Helping Professionals Involved in Counseling Others.* Unpublished master's thesis, Nell Hodgson Woodruff School of Nursing, Emory University, 1975.

Edwards, A. L. *Statistical Analysis* (revised edition). New York: Holt, Rinehart and Winston, 1958.

Eells, M. A. W. "The Research Problem," in S. D. Krampitz and N. Pavlovich (Eds.), *Readings for Nursing Research*. St. Louis: The C. V. Mosby Company, 1981.

Erikson, E. *Childhood and Society* (2nd edition). New York: W. W. Norton, 1963.

Fawcett, J. "Utilization of Nursing Research Findings," *Image*, 1982, *14*(2), pp. 57–59.

Fawcett, J. *Analysis and Evaluation of Conceptual Models of Nursing*. Philadelphia: F. A. Davis, 1984.

Fleming, J. W., and Hayter, J. "Reading Research Reports Critically," *Nursing Outlook*, 1974, *22*(3), pp. 172–175.

Fox, D. J. *Fundamentals of Research in Nursing* (4th edition). Norwalk, CN: Appleton-Century-Crofts, 1982.

Fuller, E. O. "Selecting a Clinical Nursing Problem for Research," *Image*, 1982, *14*(2), pp. 60–61.

Gaynor, J. M., Kant, D. A., and Mills, E. M. "DRGs: Regulatory and Budgetary Adjustments," *Nursing and Health Care*, 1984, *5*(5), pp. 275–279.

Good, C. V., and Scates, D. E. *Methods of Research: Educational, Psychological, Sociological*. New York: Appleton-Century-Crofts, Inc., 1954.

Gunter, L. "Literature Review," in S. D. Krampitz and N. Pavlovich (Eds.), *Readings for Nursing Research*. St. Louis: The C. V. Mosby Company, 1981.

Hallal, J. C. "The Relationship of Health Beliefs, Health Locus of Control, and Self-Concept to the Practice of Breast Self-Examination in Adult Women," *Nursing Research*, 1982, *31*(3), pp. 137–142.

Hamilton, J. M. "Nursing and DRGs: Proactive Responses to Prospective Reimbursement," *Nursing and Health Care*, 1984, *5*(3), pp. 155–159.

Hays, W. L. *Statistics*. New York: Holt, Rinehart and Winston, 1963.

Horsley, J. A., Crane, J., and Haller, K. B. *Conduct and Utilization of Research in Nursing Project*. New York: Grune & Stratton, 1981.

Huff, D. *How to Lie with Statistics*. New York: W. W. Norton & Company, Inc., 1954.

Isaac, S., and Michael, W. B. *Handbook in Research and Evaluation*. San Diego: Robert R. Knapp, Publisher, 1971.

Kerlinger, F. N. *Foundations of Behavioral Research*. New York: Holt, Rinehart and Winston, Inc., 1964.

Knapp, R. G. *Basic Statistics for Nurses*. New York: John Wiley & Sons, 1978.

Komnenich, P., and Noack, J. A. "The Process of Critiquing," in S. D. Krampitz and N. Pavlovich (Eds.), *Readings for Nursing Research*. St. Louis: The C. V. Mosby Company, 1981.

Leininger, M. M. "The Research Critique: Nature, Function, and Art," *Nursing Research*, 1968, *17*(5), pp. 444–449.

Lim-Levy, F. "The Effect of Oxygen Inhalation on Oral Temperature," *Nursing Research*, 1982, *31*(3), pp. 150–152.

Lindeman, C. A., and Schantz, D. "The Research Question," *The Journal of Nursing Administration,* 1982, January, 6–10.

Mallick, M. J. "A Constant Comparative Method for Teaching Research Critique to Baccalaureate Nursing Students," *Image,* 1983, *15*(4), pp. 120–123.

Martinson, I. M., Armstrong, G. D., Geis, D. P., Anglim, M. A., Grouseth, E. C., MacInnis, H., Nesbit, M. E., and Kersey, J. H. "Facilitating Home Care for Children Dying of Cancer," *Cancer Nursing,* 1978, *1,* pp. 41–45.

McCloskey, J. C., and Swanson, E. "Publishing Opportunities for Nurses: A Comparison of 100 Journals," *Image,* 1982, *14*(2), pp. 50–56.

Measel, C. P., and Anderson, G. C. "Nonnutritive Sucking during Tube Feedings: Effect upon Clinical Course in Premature Infants," *Journal of Obstetric, Gynecologic and Neonatal Nursing,* 1979, *8,* pp. 265–272.

Meyer, B., and Heidgerken, L. E. *Introduction to Research in Nursing.* Philadelphia: J. B. Lippincott Company, 1962.

Nightingale, F. *Notes on Nursing.* New York: Dover Publications, Inc., 1969.

The Nursing Theories Conference Group. *Nursing Theories: The Base for Nursing Practice.* Englewood Cliffs, NJ: Prentice-Hall, Inc., 1980.

Polit, D. F., and Hungler, B. P. *Nursing Research: Principles and Methods* (2nd edition). Philadelphia: J. B. Lippincott Company, 1983.

Publication Manual of the American Psychological Association (3rd edition). Washington, DC: American Psychology Association, 1983.

Riehl, J. P., and Roy, C. *Conceptual Models for Nursing Practice* (2nd edition). New York: Appleton-Century-Crofts, 1980.

Rodale, J. I. *The Synonym Finder.* Emmaus, PA: Rodale Press, 1978.

Rogers, M. E. *An Introduction to the Theoretical Basis of Nursing.* Philadelphia: F. A. Davis, 1970.

Runyon, R. P., and Haber, A. *Fundamentals of Behavioral Statistics* (2nd edition). Reading, MA: Addison-Wesley Publishing Company, 1971.

Sablay, M. C. *The Effects of a Liaison Nursing Intervention on Aftercare Compliance of Alcoholics.* Unpublished master's thesis, Nell Hodgson Woodruff School of Nursing, Emory University, 1981.

Schulz, C. M. *It's the Easter Beagle, Charlie Brown.* New York: Scholastic Book Services, 1976.

Seaman, C. C., and Verhonick, P. J. *Research Methods for Undergraduate Students in Nursing* (2nd edition). New York: Appleton-Century-Crofts, 1982.

Selye, H. *Stress of Life* (revised edition). New York: McGraw-Hill Book Company, 1976.

Siegel, S. *Nonparametric Statistics: For the Behavioral Sciences.* New York: McGraw-Hill Book Company, 1956.

Skinner, B. F. "Are Theories of Learning Necessary?" *Psychological Review,* 1950, *57,* pp. 193–216.

Stetler, C. B. *Nursing Research in a Service Setting.* Reston, VA: Reston Publishing Company, Inc., 1984.

Strauss, S. "Guidelines for Analysis of Research Reports," *The Journal of Educational Research,* 1969, *63*(4), pp. 165–169.

Strunk, W., and White, E. B. *The Elements of Style* (3rd edition). New York: Macmillan Publishing Company, Inc., 1979.

Talmadge, M. *Descriptive Study of Chemically Dependent Nurses.* Unpublished master's thesis, Nell Hodgson Woodruff School of Nursing, Emory University, 1982.

Toth, R. M. "DRGs: Imperative Strategies for Nursing Service Administration. *Nursing and Health Care,* 1984, *5*(4), pp. 197–203.

Treece, E. W., and Treece, J. W. *Elements of Research in Nursing.* St. Louis: The C. V. Mosby Company, 1982.

Waltz, C. F., and Bausell, R. B. *Nursing Research: Design, Statistics and Computer Analysis.* Philadelphia: F. A. Davis Company, 1981.

Wandelt, M. A. *Guide for the Beginning Researcher.* New York: Appleton-Century-Crofts, 1970.

Webster's New Collegiate Dictionary. Springfield, MA: G. C. Merriam Company, 1961.

APPENDIXES

APPENDIX A. Random Numbers (Two Digits)

66	27	66	87	76
85	12	91	24	22
72	54	84	19	19
63	89	22	68	31
34	29	96	94	59
50	33	36	10	85
21	88	94	34	48
46	32	83	57	21
38	31	75	48	98
75	97	78	98	96
84	79	50	39	69
71	79	54	17	94
69	19	71	19	54
86	96	10	89	73
58	17	55	52	62
19	25	57	61	10
24	82	27	99	83
21	61	15	41	72
73	52	91	82	26
81	95	96	22	93

APPENDIX B. Random Numbers (Three Digits)

762	858	122	916	245	220
729	543	847	195	190	631
897	224	686	317	344	295
962	949	599	506	331	363
107	851	214	888	942	340
487	468	328	835	575	215
382	312	751	488	987	754
975	789	987	963	847	798
505	399	695	717	791	543
177	947	691	191	719	197
542	860	968	102	894	735
581	178	552	528	625	199
250	570	617	100	245	821
277	998	836	215	615	150
412	720	733	525	918	826
264	810	956	963	226	930
801	137	506	608	446	896
267	832	577	119	382	165
162	726	692	269	579	222
187	852	952	162	115	250
930	533	116	729	975	676
877	507	189	419	716	407
655	545	493	838	308	780
637	789	430	705	207	664
774	899	677	825	303	699
939	375	865	692	640	658
289	928	135	884	100	259
677	280	869	402	318	470
483	331	845	875	738	787
538	636	661	922	650	773
854	559	420	254	867	881
400	401	389	848	617	515

APPENDIX C. Random Numbers (Four Digits)

6675	8763	7627	8589	1229	9168
2457	2206	7299	5435	8474	1954
1905	6316	8978	2247	6865	3174
3448	2958	9620	9491	5997	5060
3319	3638	1077	8512	2141	8888
9427	3405	4876	4686	3282 .	8353
5751	2157	3821	3125	7513	4880
9873	7548	9751	7899	9872	9638
8477	7988	5054	3993	6954	7170
7916	5439	1776	9479	6915	1912
7192	1978	5426	8604	9688	1024
8941	7354	5811	1784	5520	5286
6253	1999	2503	5700	6173	1003
2454	8215	2778	9984	8367	2157
6154	1502	4123	7201	7337	5285
9188	8260	2649	8103	9567	9630
2268	9309	8010	1374	5065	6080
4463	8969	2674	8323	5770	1191
3827	1659	1629	7260	6926	2691
5794	2229	1876	8520	9527	1625
1159	2508	9300	5339	1166	7297
9754	6765	8772	5071	1896	4195
7168	4076	6554	5456	4934	8381
3080	7802	6371	7897	4305	7054
2076	6642	7741	8993	6775	8253
3032	6995	9396	3759	8659	6928
6400	6589	2895	9289	1357	8843
1005	2596	6778	2804	8699	4028
3188	4707	4839	3315	8459	8751
7388	7879	5384	6367	6614	9228
6509	7734	8545	5590	4206	2542
8671	8810	4007	4011	3896	8485
6178	5155	6743	1360	7550	9295

APPENDIX D. Random Numbers (Five Digits)

66624	27534	66752	87631	76271	85890
12292	91687	24574	22069	72996	54352
84748	19548	19059	63168	89784	22477
68651	31747	34482	29589	96206	94916
59976	50600	33195	36384	10771	85120
21413	88889	94273	34059	48760	46861
32820	83530	57518	21576	38210	31258
75137	48809	98738	75486	97513	78997
98724	96381	84772	79889	50543	39939
69548	71705	79160	54394	17768	94793
69157	19121	71929	19782	54269	86045
96883	10244	89410	73545	58117	17843
55208	52861	62533	19998	25036	57003
61731	10033	24541	82152	27789	99840
83678	21572	61546	15029	41237	72010
73379	52589	91882	82607	26490	81039
95673	96305	22685	93092	80104	13748
50653	60803	44631	89692	26749	83230
57703	11911	38276	16590	16298	72604
69266	26913	57947	22298	18760	85202
95270	16258	11590	25085	93008	53391
11660	72973	97549	67651	87728	50718
18965	41951	71687	40767	65540	54562
49346	83818	30803	78023	63711	78978
43058	70548	20765	66420	77414	89932
67755	82535	30321	69953	93963	37593
86597	69284	64000	65895	28958	92897
13574	88434	10054	25967	67782	28047
86998	40284	31887	47074	48397	33151
84597	87512	73882	78798	53849	63674
66142	92284	65091	77342	85453	55906
42062	25426	86712	88100	40072	40119
38963	84854	61786	51553	67435	13609

APPENDIX E. Squares and Square Roots (Numbers 1-100)

1	1	1	51	2601	7.141429
2	4	1.414214	52	2704	7.211103
3	9	1.732051	53	2809	7.28011
4	16	2	54	2916	7.348469
5	25	2.236068	55	3025	7.416199
6	36	2.44949	56	3136	7.483315
7	49	2.645751	57	3249	7.549834
8	64	2.828427	58	3364	7.615773
9	81	3	59	3481	7.681146
10	100	3.162278	60	3600	7.745967
11	121	3.316625	61	3721	7.81025
12	144	3.464102	62	3844	7.874008
13	169	3.605551	63	3969	7.937254
14	196	3.741657	64	4096	8
15	225	3.872984	65	4225	8.062258
16	256	4	66	4356	8.124039
17	289	4.123106	67	4489	8.185353
18	324	4.242641	68	4624	8.246211
19	361	4.358899	69	4761	8.306624
20	400	4.472136	70	4900	8.3666
21	441	4.582576	71	5041	8.426149
22	484	4.690416	72	5184	8.485281
23	529	4.795832	73	5329	8.544004
24	576	4.898979	74	5476	8.602326
25	625	5	75	5625	8.660254
26	676	5.09902	76	5776	8.717798
27	729	5.196153	77	5929	8.774964
28	784	5.291503	78	6084	8.831761
29	841	5.385165	79	6241	8.888195
30	900	5.477225	80	6400	8.944272
31	961	5.567764	81	6561	9
32	1024	5.656854	82	6724	9.055386
33	1089	5.744563	83	6889	9.110434
34	1156	5.830952	84	7056	9.165151
35	1225	5.91608	85	7225	9.219544
36	1296	6	86	7396	9.273619
37	1369	6.082763	87	7569	9.327379
38	1444	6.164414	88	7744	9.380831
39	1521	6.244998	89	7921	9.433981
40	1600	6.324556	90	8100	9.486834

(Continued)

Appendix E (continued)

41	1681	6.403125	91	8281	9.539392
42	1764	6.480741	92	8464	9.591663
43	1849	6.557439	93	8649	9.64365
44	1936	6.633249	94	8836	9.69536
45	2025	6.708204	95	9025	9.746794
46	2116	6.78233	96	9216	9.797958
47	2209	6.855655	97	9409	9.848858
48	2304	6.928204	98	9604	9.899494
49	2401	7	99	9801	9.949875
50	2500	7.071068	100	10000	10

APPENDIX F. Table of Critical Values of Chi Square

Probability under H_0 that $\chi^2 \geq$ chi square

df	.99	.98	.95	.90	.80	.70	.50	.30	.20	.10	.05	.02	.01	.001
1	.00016	.00063	.0039	.016	.064	.15	.46	1.07	1.64	2.71	3.84	5.41	6.64	10.83
2	.02	.04	.10	.21	.45	.71	1.39	2.41	3.22	4.60	5.99	7.82	9.21	13.82
3	.12	.18	.35	.58	1.00	1.42	2.37	3.66	4.64	6.25	7.82	9.84	11.34	16.27
4	.30	.43	.71	1.06	1.65	2.20	3.36	4.88	5.99	7.78	9.49	11.67	13.28	18.46
5	.55	.75	1.14	1.61	2.34	3.00	4.35	6.06	7.29	9.24	11.07	13.39	15.09	20.52
6	.87	1.13	1.64	2.20	3.07	3.83	5.35	7.23	8.56	10.64	12.59	15.03	16.81	22.46
7	1.24	1.56	2.17	2.83	3.82	4.67	6.35	8.38	9.80	12.02	14.07	16.62	18.48	24.32
8	1.65	2.03	2.73	3.49	4.59	5.53	7.34	9.52	11.03	13.36	15.51	18.17	20.09	26.12
9	2.09	2.53	3.32	4.17	5.38	6.39	8.34	10.66	12.24	14.68	16.92	19.68	21.67	27.88
10	2.56	3.06	3.94	4.86	6.18	7.27	9.34	11.78	13.44	15.99	18.31	21.16	23.21	29.59
11	3.05	3.61	4.58	5.58	6.99	8.15	10.34	12.90	14.63	17.28	19.68	22.62	24.72	31.26
12	3.57	4.18	5.23	6.30	7.81	9.03	11.34	14.01	15.81	18.55	21.03	24.05	26.22	32.91
13	4.11	4.76	5.89	7.04	8.63	9.93	12.34	15.12	16.98	19.81	22.36	25.47	27.69	34.53
14	4.66	5.37	6.57	7.79	9.47	10.82	13.34	16.22	18.15	21.06	23.68	26.87	29.14	36.12
15	5.23	5.98	7.26	8.55	10.31	11.72	14.34	17.32	19.31	22.31	25.00	28.26	30.58	37.70
16	5.81	6.61	7.96	9.31	11.15	12.62	15.34	18.42	20.46	23.54	26.30	29.63	32.00	39.29
17	6.41	7.26	8.67	10.08	12.00	13.53	16.34	19.51	21.62	24.77	27.59	31.00	33.41	40.75
18	7.02	7.91	9.39	10.86	12.86	14.44	17.34	20.60	22.76	25.99	28.87	32.35	34.80	42.31
19	7.63	8.57	10.12	11.65	13.72	15.35	18.34	21.69	23.90	27.20	30.14	33.69	36.19	43.82
20	8.26	9.24	10.85	12.44	14.58	16.27	19.34	22.78	25.04	28.41	31.41	35.02	37.57	45.32
21	8.90	9.92	11.59	13.24	15.44	17.18	20.34	23.86	26.17	29.62	32.67	36.34	38.93	46.80
22	9.54	10.60	12.34	14.04	16.31	18.10	21.34	24.94	27.30	30.81	33.92	37.66	40.29	48.27
23	10.20	11.29	13.09	14.85	17.19	19.02	22.34	26.02	28.43	32.01	35.17	38.97	41.64	49.73
24	10.86	11.99	13.85	15.66	18.06	19.94	23.34	27.10	29.55	33.20	36.42	40.27	42.98	51.18
25	11.52	12.70	14.61	16.47	18.94	20.87	24.34	28.17	30.68	34.38	37.65	41.57	44.31	52.62
26	12.20	13.41	15.38	17.29	19.82	21.79	25.34	29.25	31.80	35.56	38.88	42.86	45.64	54.05
27	12.88	14.12	16.15	18.11	20.70	22.72	26.34	30.32	32.91	36.74	40.11	44.14	46.96	55.48
28	13.56	14.85	16.93	18.94	21.59	23.65	27.34	31.39	34.03	37.92	41.34	45.42	48.28	56.89
29	14.26	15.57	17.71	19.77	22.48	24.58	28.34	32.46	35.14	39.09	42.56	46.69	49.59	58.30
30	14.95	16.31	18.49	20.60	23.36	25.51	29.34	33.53	36.25	40.26	43.77	47.96	50.89	59.70

This table is taken from Table IV of Fisher and Yates, *Statistical Tables for Biological, Agricultural and Medical Research*, published by Longman Group, Ltd., London (previously published by Oliver and Boyd, Ltd., Edinburgh), and by permission of the authors and publishers.

APPENDIX G. Table of Probabilities Associated with Values as Small as Observed Values of X in the Binomial Test

Given in the body of this table are one-tailed probabilities under H_0 for the binomial test when $P = Q = \frac{1}{2}$. To save space, decimal points are omitted in the p's.

N \ x	0	1	2	3	4	5	6	7	8	9	10	11	12	13	14	15
5	031	188	500	812	969	†										
6	016	109	344	656	891	984	†									
7	008	062	227	500	773	938	992	†								
8	004	035	145	363	637	855	965	996	†							
9	002	020	090	254	500	746	910	980	998	†						
10	001	011	055	172	377	623	828	945	989	999	†					
11		006	033	113	274	500	726	887	967	994	†	†				
12		003	019	073	194	387	613	806	927	981	997	†	†			
13		002	011	046	133	291	500	709	867	954	989	998	†	†		
14		001	006	029	090	212	395	605	788	910	971	994	999	†	†	
15			004	018	059	151	304	500	696	849	941	982	996	†	†	†
16			002	011	038	105	227	402	598	773	895	962	989	998	†	†
17			001	006	025	072	166	315	500	685	834	928	975	994	999	†
18			001	004	015	048	119	240	407	593	760	881	952	985	996	999
19				002	010	032	084	180	324	500	676	820	916	968	990	998
20				001	006	021	058	132	252	412	588	748	868	942	979	994
21				001	004	013	039	095	192	332	500	668	808	905	961	987
22					002	008	026	067	143	262	416	584	738	857	933	974
23					001	005	017	047	105	202	339	500	661	798	895	953
24						001	003	011	032	076	154	271	419	581	729	846	924
25						002	007	022	054	115	212	345	500	655	788	885

† 1.0 or approximately 1.0.

This table is taken from Walker and Lev, *Statistical Inference*, published by Holt, Rinehart and Winston, 1953.

APPENDIX H. Critical Values of U and U' for a One-Tailed Test at $\alpha = 0.05$ or a Two-Tailed Test at $\alpha = 0.10$

To be significant for any given n_1 and n_2: Obtained U must be equal to or <u>less than</u> the value shown in the table. Obtained U' must be equal to or <u>greater than</u> the value shown in the table.

n_2 \ n_1	1	2	3	4	5	6	7	8	9	10	11	12	13	14	15	16	17	18	19	20
1	--	--	--	--	--	--	--	--	--	--	--	--	--	--	--	--	--	--	0	0
																			19	20
2	--	--	--	--	0	0	0	1	1	1	1	2	2	2	3	3	3	4	4	4
					10	12	14	15	17	19	21	22	24	26	27	29	31	32	34	36
3	--	--	0	0	1	2	2	3	3	4	5	5	6	7	7	8	9	9	10	11
			9	12	14	16	19	21	24	26	28	31	33	35	38	40	42	45	47	49
4	--	--	0	1	2	3	4	5	6	7	8	9	10	11	12	14	15	16	17	18
			12	15	18	21	24	27	30	33	36	39	42	45	48	50	53	56	59	62
5	--	0	1	2	4	5	6	8	9	11	12	13	15	16	18	19	20	22	23	25
		10	14	18	21	25	29	32	36	39	43	47	50	54	57	61	65	68	72	75
6	--	0	2	3	5	7	8	10	12	14	16	17	19	21	23	25	26	28	30	32
		12	16	21	25	29	34	38	42	46	50	55	59	63	67	71	76	80	84	88
7	--	0	2	4	6	8	11	13	15	17	19	21	24	26	28	30	33	35	37	39
		14	19	24	29	34	38	43	48	53	58	63	67	72	77	82	86	91	96	101
8	--	1	3	5	8	10	13	15	18	20	23	26	28	31	33	36	39	41	44	47
		15	21	27	32	38	43	49	54	60	65	70	76	81	87	92	97	103	108	113
9	--	1	3	6	9	12	15	18	21	24	27	30	33	36	39	42	45	48	51	54
		17	24	30	36	42	48	54	60	66	72	78	84	90	96	102	108	114	120	126
10	--	1	4	7	11	14	17	20	24	27	31	34	37	41	44	48	51	55	58	62
		19	26	33	39	46	53	60	66	73	79	86	93	99	106	112	119	125	132	138
11	--	1	5	8	12	16	19	23	27	31	34	38	42	46	50	54	57	61	65	69
		21	28	36	43	50	58	65	72	79	87	94	101	108	115	122	130	137	144	151
12	--	2	5	9	13	17	21	26	30	34	38	42	47	51	55	60	64	68	72	77
		22	31	39	47	55	63	70	78	86	94	102	109	117	125	132	140	148	156	163
13	--	2	6	10	15	19	24	28	33	37	42	47	51	56	61	65	70	75	80	84
		24	33	42	50	59	67	76	84	93	101	109	118	126	134	143	151	159	167	176
14	--	2	7	11	16	21	26	31	36	41	46	51	56	61	66	71	77	82	87	92
		26	35	45	54	63	72	81	90	99	108	117	126	135	144	153	161	170	179	188
15	--	3	7	12	18	23	28	33	39	44	50	55	61	66	72	77	83	88	94	100
		27	38	48	57	67	77	87	96	106	115	125	134	144	153	163	172	182	191	200

(Continued)

Appendix H (Continued)

n_1	1	2	3	4	5	6	7	8	9	10	11	12	13	14	15	16	17	18	19	20
16	--	3	8	14	19	25	30	36	42	48	54	60	65	71	77	83	89	95	101	107
		29	40	50	61	71	82	92	102	112	122	132	143	153	163	173	183	193	203	213
17	--	3	9	15	20	26	33	39	45	51	57	64	70	77	83	89	96	102	109	115
		31	42	53	65	76	86	97	108	119	130	140	151	161	172	183	193	204	214	225
18	--	4	9	16	22	28	35	41	48	55	61	68	75	82	88	95	102	109	116	123
		32	45	56	68	80	91	103	114	123	137	148	159	170	182	193	204	215	226	237
19	0	4	10	17	23	30	37	44	51	58	65	72	80	87	94	101	109	116	123	130
	19	34	47	59	72	84	96	108	120	132	144	156	167	179	191	203	214	226	238	250
20	0	4	11	18	25	32	39	47	54	62	69	77	84	92	100	107	115	123	130	138
	20	36	49	62	75	88	101	113	126	138	151	163	176	188	200	213	225	237	250	262

(Dashes in the body of the table indicate that no decision is possible at the stated level of significance.)

This table is taken from Runyon and Haber, *Fundamentals of Behavioral Statistics,* 2nd ed., published by Addison-Wesley, Inc. Reprinted by permission.

APPENDIX I. Critical Values of *t*

For any given df, the table shows the values of t corresponding to various levels of probability. Obtained t is significant at a given level if it is equal to or <u>greater than</u> the value shown in the table.

df	Level of significance for one-tailed test					
	.10	.05	.025	.01	.005	.0005
	Level of significance for two-tailed test					
	.20	.10	.05	.02	.01	.001
1	3.078	6.314	12.706	31.821	63.657	636.619
2	1.886	2.920	4.303	6.965	9.925	31.598
3	1.638	2.353	3.182	4.541	5.841	12.941
4	1.533	2.132	2.776	3.747	4.604	8.610
5	1.476	2.015	2.571	3.365	4.032	6.859
6	1.440	1.943	2.447	3.143	3.707	5.959
7	1.415	1.895	2.365	2.998	3.499	5.405
8	1.397	1.860	2.306	2.896	3.355	5.041
9	1.383	1.833	2.262	2.821	3.250	4.781
10	1.372	1.812	2.228	2.764	3.169	4.587
11	1.363	1.796	2.201	2.718	3.106	4.437
12	1.356	1.782	2.179	2.681	3.055	4.318
13	1.350	1.771	2.160	2.650	3.012	4.221
14	1.345	1.761	2.145	2.624	2.977	4.140
15	1.341	1.753	2.131	2.602	2.947	4.073
16	1.337	1.746	2.120	2.583	2.921	4.015
17	1.333	1.740	2.110	2.567	2.898	3.965
18	1.330	1.734	2.101	2.552	2.878	3.922
19	1.328	1.729	2.093	2.539	2.861	3.883
20	1.325	1.725	2.086	2.528	2.845	3.850
21	1.323	1.721	2.080	2.518	2.831	3.819
22	1.321	1.717	2.074	2.508	2.819	3.792
23	1.319	1.714	2.069	2.500	2.807	3.767
24	1.318	1.711	2.064	2.492	2.797	3.745
25	1.316	1.708	2.060	2.485	2.787	3.725
26	1.315	1.706	2.056	2.479	2.799	3.707
27	1.314	1.703	2.052	2.473	2.771	3.690
28	1.313	1.701	2.048	2.467	2.763	3.674
29	1.311	1.699	2.045	2.462	2.756	3.659
30	1.310	1.697	2.042	2.457	2.750	3.646
40	1.303	1.684	2.021	2.423	2.704	3.551
60	1.296	1.671	2.000	2.390	2.660	3.460
120	1.289	1.658	1.980	2.358	2.617	3.373
∞	1.282	1.645	1.960	2.326	2.576	3.291

This table is taken from Runyon and Haber, *Fundamentals of Behavioral Statistics,* 2nd ed., published by Addison-Wesley, Inc. Reprinted by permission.

220

APPENDIX J. Critical Values or RHO (Rank Order Correlation)

	Level of significance for one-tailed test			
	.05	.025	.01	.005
	Level of significance for two-tailed test			
n*	.10	.05	.02	.01
5	.900	1.000	1.000	—
6	.829	.886	.943	1.000
7	.714	.786	.893	.929
8	.643	.738	.833	.881
9	.600	.683	.783	.833
10	.564	.648	.746	.794
12	.506	.591	.712	.777
14	.456	.544	.645	.715
16	.425	.506	.601	.665
18	.399	.475	.564	.625
20	.377	.450	.534	.591
22	.359	.428	.508	.562
24	.343	.409	.485	.537
26	.329	.392	.465	.515
28	.317	.377	.448	.496
30	.306	.364	.432	.478

*n = number of pairs

This table is taken from Runyon and Haber, *Fundamentals of Behavioral Statistics*, 2nd ed., published by Addison-Wesley, Inc. Reprinted by permission.

APPENDIX K. Significant Values of the Correlation Coefficient

n	.1	.05	.02	.01	.001	n	.1	.05	.02	.01	.001
1	.98769	.99692	.999507	.999877	.9999988	16	.4000	.4683	.5425	.5897	.7084
2	.90000	.95000	.98000	.990000	.99900	17	.3887	.4555	.5285	.5751	.6932
3	.8054	.8783	.93433	.95873	.99116	18	.3783	.4438	.5155	.5614	.6787
4	.7293	.8144	.8822	.91720	.97406	19	.3687	.4329	.5034	.5487	.6652
5	.6694	.7545	.8329	.8745	.95074	20	.3598	.4227	.4921	.5368	.6524
6	.6215	.7067	.7887	.8343	.92493	25	.3233	.3809	.4451	.4869	.5974
7	.5822	.6664	.7498	.7977	.8982	30	.2960	.3494	.4093	.4487	.5541
8	.5494	.6319	.7155	.7646	.8721	35	.2746	.3246	.3810	.4182	.5189
9	.5214	.6021	.6851	.7348	.8471	40	.2573	.3044	.3578	.3932	.4896
10	.4973	.5760	.6581	.7079	.8233	45	.2428	.2875	.3384	.3721	.4648
11	.4762	.5529	.6339	.6835	.8010	50	.2306	.2732	.3218	.3541	.4433
12	.4575	.5324	.6120	.6614	.7800	60	.2108	.2500	.2948	.3248	.4078
13	.4409	.5139	.5923	.6411	.7603	70	.1954	.2319	.2737	.3017	.3799
14	.4259	.4973	.5742	.6226	.7420	80	.1829	.2172	.2565	.2830	.3568
15	.4124	.4821	.5577	.6055	.7246	90	.1726	.2050	.2422	.2673	.3375
						100	.1638	.1946	.2301	.2540	.3211

This table is taken from Table VII of Fisher and Yates, *Statistical Tables for Biological, Agricultural and Medical Research*, published by Longman Group, Ltd., London (previously published by Oliver and Boyd, Ltd., Edinburgh), and by permission of the authors and publishers.

INDEX

design(s)
  comparative, 56
  definition, 56
  descriptive, 68
  descriptive correlation, 70
  documentary-historical,
    68–69
  nature of experimental,
    66–68
  preexperimental, 60, 67
  pretest-posttest, 67
  quasiexperimental, 56,
    58–59, 67
  research, 1, 53, 55
  research questions, 55
  survey, 56
  and theory building, 55
  true experimental, 57, 59
developmental disabilities,
  187
developmental theory, 40
diagnostic related groups
  (GRGs), 201
dignity, 186
dilemma, definition, 184
directors of research, 202
discriminate validity, 83
discussion, 136–42
  critique of, 179
  example, 139–41
  example critiqued, 141–42
dispersion, 102
dissertation, 8
distribution, 116
distribution curve, 111
documentary-historical design,
  68–69
documentation of care, 201
drugs, 185
dying children, home care,
  199

economic value of research,
  198
effect variables, 46
element, information, 186
emotions, measurement of,
  50
enumeration data, 94
environmental factors, as
  source of errors, 85
environmental variables, 44, 51
equipment, 84
equivalence, 83
error, type I and II, 110–11
errors, sources of, 85

ethical
  considerations, 10, 181,
    183–84
  dilemmas, 181, 192
  issues, 191–93
  responsibility, 184, 192
  theories, 188–89
examples
  abstract, 160–61, 165–66
  conclusions, 145–46
  discussion, 139–41
  ethical issues in research,
    191–93
  preexperimental design, 60
  presentation of analysis of
    data, 132–33
  presentation of data, 129–30
  presentation of findings,
    125–27
  recommendations, 148–49
  research question, formula-
    tion of, 13–14
  review of literature, 22–28
  summary, 143–44
expected value, in chi square,
  105
experimental approaches, 56,
  57
experimental design, 58–59,
  66–68
experimental drug, 189
experimental group, 112,
  117–18
experimental studies, 56–57
experimental variable, 45
expert, 181
extraneous variables, 44,
  51–52

F test, 116
face validity, 83–84
facts, 124
Fagin, C., 198–200
falsity, 117
feasibility, quasiexperimental,
  59
federal guidelines, 183
fetus research, 184
fidelity to promises and contracts, 189
findings, 24, 123–24, 189, 191
  assumptions, 136
  communicating, 6
  critique of, 179
  inconclusive, 123, 138–39
  interpretation of, 136–42

findings (*cont.*)
  maximize, 181
  opposite direction, 137–38
  order of presentation, 124
  predicted direction, 136–37
  presentation of, 1, 124
  recommendations, 148
  relevance of, 181
  of research reviewed, 20
  serendipitous, 123, 135–36
  significant, 123
  theory and literature, 137
Fisher exact probability test,
  98
formulation
  of hypotheses, 48
  of research question, 3,
    13–14
framework, theoretical, 177
fraud, 191
frequencies, 94
frequency, 97, 99–102
frequency data, 94, 112
frequency distribution, 100
Friedman 2-way ANOVA, 98

Gaussian distribution, 116
generalizability, of research
  tool, 80
generalization, 8, 52, 58, 65,
  66, 70, 146
  preexperimental design, 60
  quasiexperimental design,
    59
generalizations, subject considerations, 20
generation of information, preexperimental design, 60
"good" client, 186
goods, distribution of, 190
gratitude, for benefits received, 189
guardians, 187

Hawthorne effect, 68
health care costs, 198
health promotion, 182, 190
historical design, example, 71
historical research, 70
history
  preexperimental design, 60
  quasiexperimental design,
    59
homogeneity
  in research tools, 83
  of variance, 89, 99, 116

THE
REAL
WIN

Pursuing God's Plan
for Authentic Success

MEN'S BIBLE STUDY

COLT McCOY
MATT CARTER

LifeWay Press®
Nashville, Tennessee

Published by LifeWay Press®
© 2013 Colt McCoy and Matt Carter
Published by arrangement with The Waterbrook Multnomah
Publishing Group, a division of Random House Inc.
Reprinted December 2016

ISBN 978-1-4158-7794-4
Item 005558786

Dewey decimal classification: 248.842
Subject headings: HUNTING \ MEN \ OUTDOOR RECREATION

Unless indicated otherwise, all Scripture quotations are taken from The Holy Bible, English Standard
Version, copyright © 2000, 2001 by Crossway Bibles, a division of Good News Publishers. Scripture
quotations marked NIV are taken from the Holy Bible, NEW INTERNATIONAL VERSION®. Copyright
© 1973, 1978, 1984 by Biblica Inc. All rights reserved worldwide. Used by permission. Scripture
quotations marked NASB are taken from the New American Standard Bible®, Copyright © 1960,
1962, 1963, 1968, 1971, 1972, 1973, 1975, 1977, 1995 by TheLockman Foundation. Used by permission.
(www.lockman.org)

To order additional copies of this resource, write to LifeWay Church Resources Customer Service; One
LifeWay Plaza; Nashville, TN 37234-0113; fax 615.251.5933; phone toll free 800.458.2772; order online
at www.lifeway.com; email orderentry@lifeway.com; or visit the LifeWay Christian Store serving you.

Printed in the United States of America

Adult Ministry Publishing
LifeWay Church Resources
One LifeWay Plaza
Nashville, TN 37234-0152

CONTENTS

THE AUTHORS

COLT McCOY is an NFL quarterback. As a college player at the University of Texas, he was the most winning quarterback in the history of NCAA football, leading the Longhorns to the 2010 BCS national-championship game. During his senior year Colt won 13 of the top 15 major college-player awards, including quarterback of the year, offensive player of the year, and outstanding football player of the year. He was also a 2008 Heisman trophy runner-up. Colt has been involved in domestic and international ministries. He and his wife, Rachel, live in Austin, Texas. For more information visit *www.coltmccoy.com.*

MATT CARTER serves as the pastor of preaching and vision at Austin Stone Community Church in Austin, Texas. Planted in 2002, the church has grown from a core team of 15 to more than 8,000 regular attendees today. Matt holds a master's degree in divinity from Southwestern Seminary and is pursuing a doctorate of ministry from Southeastern Seminary. He is a coauthor of *For the City* and of the LifeWay Bible studies *Creation Unraveled* and *Creation Restored.* Matt and his wife, Jennifer, live in Austin with their three children. For more information visit *www.austinstone.org.*

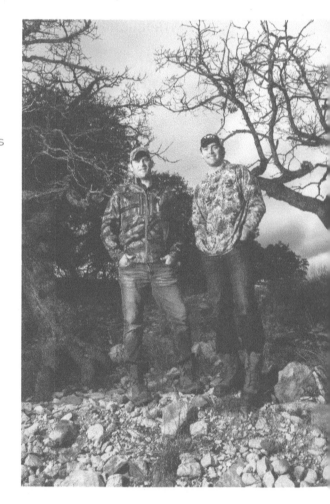

ACKNOWLEDGMENTS

MATT: I'd like to thank Marcus Brotherton, Jordan Bazant, Travis Wussow, David Kopp, and Stephen Crawford. It would have been impossible to write this book without all of you. I'd also like to thank the elders, staff, and partners of Austin Stone Community Church. Partnering with you for the sake of the gospel has been one of the greatest joys of my life.

COLT: I'd like to thank my wife, Rachel; my parents, Brad and Debra; and Jordan Bazant. A huge thanks to Gary and Blair Schwarz and their family for opening up the Tecomate Ranch for us to film and for all their help with the project. We also want to thank Robert and Susan Patterson and their family for their incredible generosity and hospitality in opening up the Texas Mountain Ranch for us to film. This project literally couldn't have been done without these families' generosity.

AIM FOR THE BEST

1. Attend each group experience.

- Watch the DVD teaching.

- Participate in the group discussion.

2. Complete the content in this workbook.

- Read the lessons and complete the learning activities.

- Memorize each week's suggested memory verse.

- Be honest with God, yourself, and others about your failures and successes as a man.

- Ask God to help you become a man who pursues the real win in life.

3. Consider going deeper into the topics in this study.

- Obtain and read the book *The Real Win* by Colt McCoy and Matt Carter (Multnomah, 2013, ISBN 978-1-6014-2482-2).

INTRODUCTION

If you're like most men, you've tasted success at different points in your life. You've set goals and achieved them. You've put your nose to the grindstone and worked day after day to see different dreams come true. Sure, things may not be going exactly as you planned right now, but there have been moments in the game of your life when you felt you were playing well and taking the lead.

In other words, you know what it's like to win.

And yet, if you're like most men, you've also felt a nagging sense that what you're working so hard to achieve might not be the right goal after all. You do your best at work and at home, but there are times when you can't stop feeling you've got your ladder leaning against the wrong wall.

We've felt the same way. Both of us have experienced moments of victory that were amazing—honestly. And yet both of us have stumbled through more than our share of failures in our efforts to win at life in a way that really counts.

That's why we've written this study—because we've discovered there's a real win out there for each of us. There's a real win out there for you. There's a way to live and love and work and play that feels genuine instead of hollow. And it's a way that allows us to become the men we were truly created to be.

We don't promise that everything will be rosy, because it won't. You'll still fail, as we did. You'll have to learn some things the hard way, as we still do.

But we can promise the teaching in this study is based on biblical principles and the more you learn to pursue God's way of doing things, the more your definition of *success* will change and grow in the most important areas of your life. In other words, your quest for authentic success can start here. We call it the real win.

If you want that kind of life—that kind of win—then keep reading.

THE
REAL WIN

WELCOME
TO THIS GROUP DISCUSSION OF *THE REAL WIN.*

OPENING ACTIVITY. To facilitate introductions and highlight the theme of this study, spend a few minutes as a group playing a round of Flip. Find a partner and take turns flipping a coin. The person who isn't flipping the coin should call heads or tails while the coin is in the air, and that person is awarded a point if the call is correct. No points are awarded or deducted for an incorrect call. After five flips the partner with the most points is declared the winner.

Use the following questions to debrief the activity.

- Did you care whether you won the game of Flip? Why or why not?

- What do you like best about winning games or challenges?

- What emotions do you typically experience when you lose?

What ideas or images come to mind when you hear the word *success*?

How can people determine whether they've achieved success in life?

To prepare to watch the DVD segment, read aloud the following verses.

> After a long time the master of those servants came and settled accounts with them. And he who had received the five talents came forward, bringing five talents more, saying, "Master, you delivered to me five talents; here I have made five talents more." His master said to him, "Well done, good and faithful servant. You have been faithful over a little; I will set you over much. Enter into the joy of your master."
> **MATTHEW 25:19-21**

WATCH DVD session 1.

DISCUSS the DVD segment with your group, using the following questions.

What did you like best about the visual elements in the DVD segment?

What did you like best about the discussion between Colt and Matt? Why?

Describe some of your favorite hobbies and interests as a child.

How have you been influenced by those hobbies and interests as you've grown into adulthood?

What steps have you recently taken to prepare for success in this life?

Respond to Matt's statement: "The Bible's definition of *success* is not achieving the goal, but the Bible's definition of *success* is being faithful in the little things that God gives you."

Colt mentioned that he's always struggled with losing. What obstacles prevent you from more consistently serving God with the little things He's given you?

APPLICATION. Throughout the week keep an eye open for the gifts God has given you in this life. Make a list (mental or physical) of the little opportunities you encounter to serve Him faithfully in the little things.

THIS WEEK'S SCRIPTURE MEMORY. Isaiah 26:4:

> Trust in the LORD forever,
> for the LORD GOD is an everlasting rock.

ASSIGNMENT. Read week 1 and complete the activities before the next group experience.

What Is **Success**?

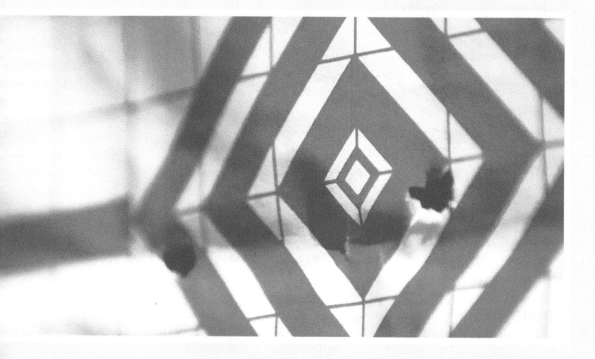

When it comes to the game of life, many of us are aiming at different targets. We have many different definitions of what it means to be successful in this world.

For example, success might be—

- landing a great job and rising to the top of your field;

- attracting the hottest, most understanding wife possible;

- living a life full of excitement and adventure;

- making a ton of money and feeling financially secure;

- gaining power and influence over people and large portions of the culture;

- being respected by others;

- doing something important and changing the world for the better.

These examples of success reflect the most popular values in our culture; they surround us every day. Do you see the ultimate goal of your life represented in the list? Or are you aiming at a different target when you live and work each day—a different purpose?

We'll begin this study by redefining *success* in a way that's significantly different from the previous examples; we'll look at success from God's perspective. In doing so, we'll gain a better understanding of what it means to serve God faithfully and to trust Him with our lives. And through it all we'll start to discover what the real win is all about.

WRESTLING WITH SUCCESS

COLT'S STORY

My whole life I've been hardwired to win. My dad was a successful coach for more than 25 years, so I learned early on that there's a pretty fine line between winning and losing, success and failure. I also learned early on that I don't like to lose.

Now if you're a boy growing up in Texas with a football in your hands, chances are good that you dream of playing at the University of Texas, leading your team to victory during the national championship, and winning the Heisman Trophy to be recognized as the best college football player in the country. That's the ultimate victory for someone like me.

I came so close.

During my senior year in 2009 I was the starting quarterback for the University of Texas Longhorns. We had a great team, and we'd had a great season by the time I traveled to New York City for the presentation of the Heisman Trophy. This was my second year as a finalist for the award, and I felt that I had a good chance to win.

In the closest points race since 1985, I came in third. Not bad, but the bottom line was that I didn't win. Part of my chance for ultimate victory was gone.

Still, we had the national championship to play for—another chance to accomplish the dream I'd been pushing for my whole life. We were the underdogs against the University of Alabama Crimson Tide, but I was confident we could win. I'd played with my teammates for four years at that point, and I knew what we were capable of. We'd trained together for weeks, and I'd never felt more prepared than I did going into that game.

Part of that preparation was spiritual, and that's how I came across Isaiah 26:3-4 during my devotions in the days leading up to the national championship:

> You keep him in perfect peace
> whose mind is stayed on you,
> because he trusts in you.
> Trust in the LORD forever,
> for the LORD GOD is an everlasting rock.

That's the text I meditated on as I took the field for the biggest game of my life, and it's become the passage that undergirds what my life is about today.

The game itself couldn't have started out much better for my team and me. Our defense intercepted the ball from Alabama, and our offense drove right down the field. I completed several passes in a row and was trying to run for a score when I got hit by a three-hundred-pound defensive lineman and felt something go wrong with my right shoulder—my throwing shoulder.

It wasn't a huge hit. I'd taken a lot worse over the years, and I wanted to bounce right up and try again for that touchdown. But my right arm was numb from the shoulder to my fingers; I couldn't raise it or grip the ball. I was in shock as I jogged over to the sideline and talked with our trainers. I wanted to get back on the field!

But I never did. The trainers worked to get me back in shape while my backup, a freshman, did his best to lead our offense. Eventually, I was taken to the locker room to confirm the worst: my arm wasn't getting better anytime soon. I sat on the bench for the rest of the game and watched as my team fought valiantly. In the end, though, we lost.

My dream was dead.

Walking off the field after the game, I felt more disappointed than at any other point in my life. That's when the sideline reporter for ABC tugged on my jersey and asked for an interview. I nodded, and she asked the question I knew was coming: "Colt, what was it like for you to watch this game—the last game in uniform—from the sideline?"

I didn't know what to say, so I started by talking about my passion for the game of football and about how much I wanted to get back on the field. I congratulated Alabama on its victory and praised my team for fighting hard.

Then I said something that still surprises me to this day: "I always give God the glory. I never question why things happen the way they do. God is in control of my life, and I know that if nothing else, I'm standing on the Rock."

I know those words came to me because of God. Yes, they came partly because I'd been meditating on Isaiah 26:3-4 before the game, but there was more to it. During the most difficult and disappointing moment of my life, God gave me peace. Something clicked into place, and I truly understood that God was my Rock and that my life wouldn't be shattered, no matter how many dreams I failed to achieve.

I realized that God was in control, and He would always be in control.

> What were some of your most ambitious dreams as a child?
> Record three.
> 1.
> 2.
> 3.
>
> How do you typically respond to disappointment?
>
>
>
> Look again at Isaiah 26:3-4. What does it mean that God
> is "an everlasting rock" (v. 4)?

REDEFINING *SUCCESS*

One of the nice things about sports is that it's pretty easy to figure out whether you're winning or losing. If you're playing football and your team has more points than the other team, you're winning. If you're running a race and you see someone running in front of you, you're losing. It's simple.

Unfortunately, real life is more complicated. Most men like to win as often as possible, but when it comes to everyday life, there are no specific measures that tell us whether we're ahead of the game or behind.

For example, think through the following list of circumstances men commonly face in today's society. Is it even possible to pinpoint what winning looks like for each one?

- A married man wants to be a good husband to his wife.

- A single man longs to have a loving wife and family.

- A man is struggling with a particular sin and wants to be free.

- A younger man is looking for a satisfying career.

- A father wants to be a good role model for his children.

- An older man is dissatisfied with his job and wants to feel fulfilled.

- A father is preparing for his child to leave home.

    Circle any of the previous situations that directly apply to you.

What would you consider to be a win for the situations you circled?

Here's the point: all men define *success* in their own ways. They all have dreams they're shooting for and goals they're trying to achieve. But are they the right dreams? Are they the correct goals? How can anyone know?

We've written this study because both of us have tried to come up with our own versions of success in this life, and we've both failed. You'll hear more about those failures—and the lessons we learned from them—in the pages to come. Thankfully, all of the times we've missed the mark have helped us gain a better understanding of what authentic success looks like for men who are attempting to follow Christ.

On a scale of 1 to 10, how confident are you that you're winning the game of your life?

1	2	3	4	5	6	7	8	9	10
Not confident									Fully confident

How would you define success in life?

The concept of the real win is built on two simple but strategic components: whom you serve and whom you trust. Those two decisions change everything for a man, and we'll take a deeper look at each one this week.

What we need you to understand now is that pursuing the real win may require you to redefine your definition of *success*. It may require you to change your understanding of what it means to win by exploring what success looks like through the lens of the Bible rather than through the lenses of our culture or your own desires.

Are you willing to do that? Pursuing the real win takes resolve, and the decision to shoot for it is a choice you make more than once. It requires courage, faith, and determination—and it certainly isn't always easy.

But take it from two guys who've been knocked down a few times and learned a few things: it's worth it.

WHY FAITHFULNESS IS KEY

The real win in this life is built on two simple ideas: whom you serve and whom you trust. You've probably figured out that God should be the *whom* in both of those phrases. People can find authentic success in life only when they commit to serve God and trust Him.

But what does that actually mean for guys like us? What does it look like to serve God every day? Why should we trust Him, and how do we go about it?

> **What ideas or images come to mind when you think of serving God?**

> **What does it mean to trust God?**

Let's start by taking a deeper look at what it means for us to serve God as men in search of the real win.

FAITHFUL IN SMALL THINGS

In the Bible a good place to start exploring the concept of serving God is Jesus' parable of the talents in Matthew 25. If you're not familiar with that story, a rich guy went on a long journey. Before he left, he gave different sums of money to three of his servants in order to keep his business rolling. The first guy got five talents, the second guy got two talents, and the third guy got one talent. A talent was payment for six thousand days of work, so each servant received a lot of money.

The first two servants immediately got to work and started investing the money they'd been given. But the third servant took a different approach. He decided to hide the money by digging a hole and burying it.

Here's what happened next:

> After a long time the master of those servants came and settled
> accounts with them. And he who had received the five talents came
> forward, bringing five talents more, saying, "Master, you delivered to
> me five talents; here I have made five talents more." His master said to
> him, "Well done, good and faithful servant. You have been faithful over
> a little; I will set you over much. Enter into the joy of your master."
> **MATTHEW 25:19-21**

Notice that the word *faithful* pops up a couple times. That's an important concept
to keep in mind when it comes to serving God. Here's the dictionary definition:

> Faithful: (1) strict or thorough in the performance of duty:
> a faithful worker; (2) true to one's word, promises, vows, etc.;
> (3) steady in allegiance or affection; loyal; constant.[1]

What friends and family members would you describe as faithful? Why?

Would your friends and family describe you as faithful? Why or why not?

The second servant got the same praise as the first one. But the third didn't fare
so well. He dug up the talent he'd been given, wiped off the dirt, and brought it
back. He said he'd been afraid because the master was a "hard man" (v. 24), and
he didn't want to risk losing anything. So he'd done nothing with the money. Not
surprisingly, the master wasn't impressed:

> His master answered him, "You wicked and slothful servant! You knew
> that I reap where I have not sown and gather where I scattered no
> seed? Then you ought to have invested my money with the bankers,
> and at my coming I should have received what was my own with
> interest. So take the talent from him and give it to him who has the
> ten talents. For to everyone who has will more be given, and he will
> have an abundance. But from the one who has not, even what he has
> will be taken away. And cast the worthless servant into the outer
> darkness. In that place there will be weeping and gnashing of teeth."
> **MATTHEW 25:26-30**

What's the difference between the first two servants and the third servant? Faithfulness. The first two servants had been given resources, and they faithfully served their master by using those resources to do the work their master wanted done. The third servant focused on himself rather than his master. He didn't want to work; he didn't want to take risks. So he did nothing. He was unfaithful.

Here's the point: authentic success in this life means being faithful with the little things God gives us. We find the real win by serving God and doing His work with whatever resources we've got.

> **What are some of the main resources you've been given that could be used to serve God and do His work on earth?**

> **Which of these resources are being wasted on pursuits that don't have eternal significance?**

> **What steps could you take this week to make better use of one or two of those resources?**

We'll keep digging into this concept as we move through the study and focus on key pursuits such as leadership, work, family, and so on. For now, though, notice how the first two servants were rewarded. When they faithfully served with a few resources, they were given more resources—not to get fat and happy with but to continue serving and doing their master's work on a larger scale.

The same can be true of us. When we're faithful to serve God with whatever He's given us, He will give us greater opportunities to serve faithfully and do the work of His kingdom.

Fill in the blank for this statement: "If only I had more _____,
I could make a real difference in my community."

What steps can you take to approach God about that missing resource?

FAITHFUL AT ALL TIMES

We just talked about the good news: we can experience the real win as men
by faithfully serving God with the little things He gives us. And as we're faithful
in those small things, He will give us a chance to be faithful with bigger things.
That's authentic success.

Now here's the bad news: it won't be smooth sailing for any of us. We'll all go
through tough times and difficult circumstances—even if we're serving God.

If you don't agree, just look at these words from the apostle Paul:

> Five times I received at the hands of the Jews the forty lashes less
> one. Three times I was beaten with rods. Once I was stoned. Three
> times I was shipwrecked; a night and a day I was adrift at sea; on
> frequent journeys, in danger from rivers, danger from robbers,
> danger from my own people, danger from Gentiles, danger in the
> city, danger in the wilderness, danger at sea, danger from false
> brothers; in toil and hardship, through many a sleepless night, in
> hunger and thirst, often without food, in cold and exposure.
> **2 CORINTHIANS 11:24-27**

Whoa! Paul was describing just some of the hardships he'd been through in his
efforts to serve God and spread the gospel message. He did the right thing, and
he still faced all kinds of adversity. The same will be true for us.

How have you experienced tough times in the past year?

How did those tough times affect the way you used your resources
in serving God?

The big challenge for us as men is to continue faithfully serving God even when
things get tough. We need to keep working and keep the right focus even when
challenges knock us down, even when we feel disappointed or discouraged, and
even when we don't understand what's going on.

What helps you stay focused on a challenging task?

How do you stay focused on God during a challenging time?

When we can serve God and be faithful with the little things despite the troubles in
our lives, we'll hear the same words the first two servants heard:

> Well done, good and faithful servant. You have been faithful over
> a little; I will set you over much. Enter into the joy of your master.
> **MATTHEW 25:23**

We'll be able to say what Paul said near the end of his life:

> I have fought the good fight, I have finished the race, I have kept the
> faith. Henceforth there is laid up for me the crown of righteousness,
> which the Lord, the righteous judge, will award to me on that Day,
> and not only to me but also to all who have loved his appearing.
> **2 TIMOTHY 4:7-8**

That's the real win.

FAITHFULNESS AND YOU

MATT'S STORY

I have vivid memories of the night I began to feel massive pains in the pit of my stomach, completely out of the blue. I was taken to the hospital and was told I needed an emergency appendectomy. The operation went well. I stayed overnight to be safe, and then I went home. Problem solved.

Or so I thought. A couple days later I was sitting at my desk at work when I got a phone call from my wife. She'd heard from the doctor. They'd found a malignant tumor in my appendix after the operation. I had cancer.

It turned out to be a carcinoid tumor of the appendix, which is a fairly rare type of cancer. Such tumors typically start to spread either when they become 2.0 centimeters long or when they break through the appendix wall. My tumor was 1.9 centimeters long and had already broken through the wall, so this was bad.

Doctors also told me that if this type of cancer spreads into your lymph nodes, you're done. Chemo doesn't work. Radiation doesn't work. It's a slow-growing cancer, so it takes a few years to kill you. And there's no hope.

I'll spare you the gory details of all my tests, but the upshot was that my blood levels came back abnormally high, and my lymph nodes had swollen significantly— a double dose of bad news. It looked as if the cancer had already spread.

The other possibility was that my blood markers were high because of the original tumor and that my lymph nodes were swollen because of the surgery. The only way to know for sure was to wait a few months and see whether anything changed, but I could tell the doctors were less than hopeful. Chances were slim that it would turn out all right.

As a 31-year-old man, I was preparing to die.

For the next three months I sat on pins and needles, thinking, hoping, and praying. I experienced every dark emotion imaginable. What would happen to my wife and children? What would happen to my church? I struggled to understand why God would allow this to happen to me.

During the darkest of those days, a friend pointed me to Psalm 39:4-5. He'd been praying for me, and he felt that God wanted to speak to me through that passage:

> Show me, O LORD, my life's end
> and the number of my days;
> let me know how fleeting is my life.
> You have made my days a mere handbreadth;
> the span of my years is as nothing before you.
> Each man's life is but a breath (NIV).

I chewed on those verses awhile. Have you ever breathed on a window on a cold winter's day? It fogs up, but then the fog instantly disappears. That's what David was saying a man's life is like—here for a brief moment, then gone. David knew that when a man grasps how short his life is, he begins to live with a new sense of what's truly important.

God was showing me there's a direct connection between understanding how short my life is and the urgency with which I'd live that life. God wanted to teach me how to number my days, how to know time was short, and how not to live in vain. God wanted me to live with holy urgency. That was a tough lesson to learn, and I was still missing an essential ingredient: trust.

The night before my next round of tests—the ones that would tell me whether I'd live or die—I paced around my bedroom and vented to my wife, Jennifer, about how frustrated I felt. Anxious and exhausted, I yelled, "What does God want from me? I've done everything I can think of. What's He trying to teach me?"

Calmly, my wife looked at me and said, "Matt, I don't know what God's trying to teach you. But I know this: He wants you to *trust Him.*"

The next day I went to the cancer ward and sat in the waiting room, surrounded by dying people. My Bible in my hands, I began reading the account of Jesus on the cross. As I read, I realized that Jesus fully trusted God even while He was being tortured and crucified. The cross didn't look like a win for someone who was going to save the world. Yet the cross was exactly what God had planned for Jesus. The nails were in Jesus' hands for a reason.

Something turned in my heart, and it hit me like a bolt of lightning: sometimes trusting God means you don't get to climb down from your cross. Whatever difficulty you're bearing, whatever goal you're not achieving, staying in that difficulty might be a part of God's perfect plan for your life.

In other words, losing in the eyes of the world might be success in the eyes of God.

After my second round of tests, I went back to my office, got on my knees, and prayed, "Lord, if it's Your will for me to die, I trust You." I'd said this to Him before, but this was the first time I really meant it. I fully surrendered right then. I let go. A peace and confidence came over me as I'd never felt before. Without a shadow of a doubt, I knew that every moment of my life was in God's hands.

The next day a phone call came. My blood work was normal. My lymph nodes were normal. All of my test results were normal. There was no sign of cancer anywhere. As of the writing of this book, I've been completely cancer-free for seven years.

Now I don't know if God miraculously healed me or if I'd never had any other cancer besides the appendix tumor. And I'm not saying that if you trust God, He will solve your problems the way my cancer was taken away from me. But this is what I know for sure: God brought me to a place where I said, "If You want to keep me on the cross, then I trust You." And I still do.

Who are some people you trust most in this life? Why do you trust them?

What are some obstacles that prevent you from trusting people?

CHOOSE TO TRUST

We've made the case that authentic success isn't about big achievements and flashy victories in this life. Rather, the real win means faithfully serving God in the little things, especially when the going gets tough. But how? How can we stay faithful and keep serving when we feel beaten down or afraid—when we don't even understand what God wants from us?

The answer is trust. You can't serve God—you can't be faithful with the resources He's given you—unless you trust Him.

How much do you trust God with the details of your life?

1   2   3   4   5   6   7   8   9   10

I don't trust Him.   I fully trust Him.

What obstacles prevent you from trusting God more?

We wish we could give you some easy advice on that subject. You know, seven steps to build your trust in God. But in the end, trust mostly comes down to a choice. After all, how do you develop trust in a human being? You decide whether that person is trustworthy, and then you choose to act based on that belief.

The same is true with God. He's completely and perfectly trustworthy: "God is faithful, by whom you were called into the fellowship of his Son, Jesus Christ our Lord" (1 Cor. 1:9). If you believe God is the all-powerful Creator of the universe—if you believe He cares for you, if you believe Jesus sacrificed Himself on the cross so that you can be saved—you must choose to take actions that confirm your belief. In other words, you must choose to trust Him, and your trust will result in actions that you take by faith.

We want so badly to succeed as men. We want to reach our goals and find victory while we fight the good fight. But here's the big question: If you don't achieve your hopes and dreams in life, can you still trust God?

What's your answer to the previous question?

How can you actively demonstrate trust in God this week? What choices will you make, and what actions will you take?

As you'll see in the weeks to come, this study is all about trusting God in the deepest way possible. This is where the real win comes from in a man's life. You can trust God because He's always faithful.

1. "Faithful," *Dictionary.com* [online, cited 1 April 2013]. Available from the Internet: *http://dictionary.reference.com*.

LEADERSHIP

WELCOME BACK
TO THIS GROUP DISCUSSION OF *THE REAL WIN.*

The previous session's application activity challenged you to list the opportunities you experienced to serve God faithfully in the little things. If you're comfortable, talk about your experiences and your list.

Describe what you liked best about the study material in week 1. What questions do you have?

ACTIVITY. Work together as a group to make a list of the best leaders you can think of from your lifetime—men and women who've made a significant impact in our culture by leading others. (If possible, ask a volunteer to record the list on a whiteboard or on a sheet of paper.) Once you have between 10 and 20 names on the list, discuss the following questions to debrief the experience.

- What are some common characteristics displayed by the leaders on your list?

- What are some leadership styles represented by the leaders on your list?

- As a group, work to define the concept of leadership in a single sentence.

To prepare to watch the DVD segment, read aloud the following verses.

> God said, "Let us make man in our image, after our likeness. And let
> them have dominion over the fish of the sea and over the birds of
> the heavens and over the livestock and over all the earth and over
> every creeping thing that creeps on the earth." So God created
> man in his own image, in the image of God he created him; male
> and female he created them. And God blessed them. And God said
> to them, "Be fruitful and multiply and fill the earth and subdue it,
> and have dominion over the fish of the sea and over the birds of the
> heavens and over every living thing that moves on the earth."
> **GENESIS 1:26-28**

WATCH DVD session 2.

DISCUSS the DVD segment with your group, using the following questions.

What did you like best about the visual elements in the DVD segment?

What did you like best about the discussion between Colt and Matt? Why?

In what areas of life do others look to you as a leader?

What have you learned about the practice and responsibility of leadership from the example of your parents?

Respond to Matt's statement: "[To be a leader] is not a position; it's a role that requires action."

Matt and Colt defined *leadership* as the choice "to do what's right even when it's not popular and even when it's not easy." When have you recently had to make difficult choices as a leader?

How should we move forward when we fail to lead well in different areas?

APPLICATION. We serve best as leaders in our families and workplaces when we're actively following Jesus Christ, the only perfect leader who's ever lived. Commit to study a portion of God's Word every day in the coming week and to spend time in prayer when you need to make important decisions as a leader. Be prepared to talk about these experiences during the next session.

THIS WEEK'S SCRIPTURE MEMORY. 1 Corinthians 11:3:

> I want you to understand that the head of every man is Christ,
> the head of a wife is her husband, and the head of Christ is God.

ASSIGNMENT. Read week 2 and complete the activities before the next group experience.

You Are a Leader

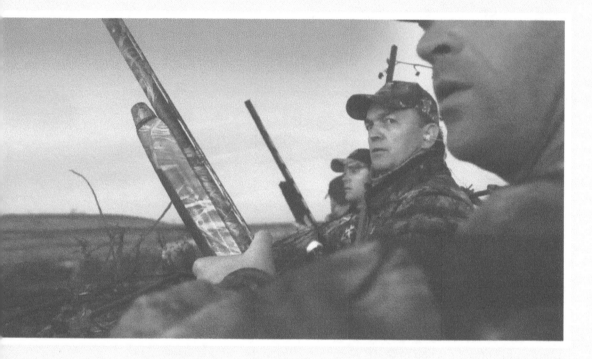

There are lots of leaders in today's society, and there are lots of different titles and descriptions we use to label leaders. Here are just a few: coach, boss, president, parent, manager, captain, and so on.

Have you worn one of those labels in the past? Are you wearing one of those labels now? If so, you're a leader. And even if you haven't held an official position that forced people to follow you, there's another leadership label we need to add to the list: man.

That's right. If you're a man, you're called to be a leader.

If you're a husband, you're called to lead your wife. If you're a father, you're called to lead your children. If you have a job, live in a community, or attend a church, you're called to be a witness for God's kingdom and lead within those areas of influence.

Does that mean women shouldn't be leaders or aren't qualified to have positions of influence in today's culture? No, we're not saying that. Women can be gifted leaders too.

But as we'll see this week, the Bible makes it clear that *all* men are called to lead. All men are leaders, so it's important for all men to understand what leadership means and how they can fulfill their roles in God's kingdom.

CALLED TO LEAD

COLT'S STORY

I know what it's like to lead. I also know what it's like to struggle with the weight and responsibility of leadership.

As a quarterback, I strive to be a leader on my team both on and off the field. That's a skill I've cultivated over the years—in high school, in college, and now in the NFL. I strive to set a high standard for myself, and I ask my teammates to follow.

But things are a little different for me as a new husband. I'm still learning my responsibilities in that arena—what I'm supposed to do, what I can do, and what I should never do. I've found it can be harder to lead a marriage than an NFL team!

In my first season with the Cleveland Browns, Matt and Jennifer came to visit my wife, Rachel, and me. I was going through a rough patch in my job. We were playing well as a football team, but we were still losing. Matt and Jenn came to our game against the St. Louis Rams. In the last few minutes of the game, our team drove the ball all the way downfield to set up a game-winning field goal. But because of a rare misplaced snap, our kicker missed the field goal, and we lost.

Later that night I was feeling pretty low as the four of us talked together. I kept asking whether it was all worth it—the punishment, pain, and scrutiny of being in the spotlight all the time. Rachel confessed to Matt and Jenn how hard it was to see me depressed like that. It's not easy for a young wife to see her husband so down, and this wasn't the first time I'd been this way. My attitude was difficult on our marriage, the stress was taking a toll, and we were finding it difficult to connect with each other in the midst of it all.

I've since learned that difficult circumstances are the exact times when a man needs to lead.

Recently, Matt and Jenn came back for another visit, this time in the summer. I'd done some good thinking and praying since the last time they'd seen us, but my job was still difficult. In fact, the Browns had drafted another quarterback only a few months earlier, and I was working hard to keep my job as a starter.

Because of the hours I was putting into training, I wasn't doing a great job of communicating well with the people I loved.

Matt and Jenn were worried, so they came to see us. One evening while I was still at the training facility, Jenn asked my wife, "How is Colt doing? And be honest."

Rachel said, "Honestly, it's been great. Colt's been a different man this year compared to what was happening inside him last year. His job is still incredibly stressful, but he's changing as a man and husband. Now he comes home and makes a conscious effort to be present. The only thing I can figure out is that God has done a good work in his heart."

She was right. I'd been spending a lot of time with God, and He'd been helping me redefine my views of success. I had a better understanding of what was important and what wasn't, and I was learning to be faithful in serving Him (and the people closest to me) even when things were disappointing with my job.

Matt later told me how happy he was to hear about those changes. He could see that God was working on my heart and that I was responding to His call for me to lead well at home. I was learning to live not as an immature guy but as a mature man seeking authentic success.

Again, the change wasn't due to anything special in me. It was all thanks to God's work in my life.

What ideas or images come to mind when you hear the word *leader?*

Who among your friends and family do you consider a good leader? Record three examples and include what attributes help each person lead well.

1.

2.

3.

When have you recently been asked to lead in a specific area?
What happened?

BORN LEADERS

A TV sitcom featured an episode in which a teenage girl and her boyfriend discovered they were going to have a baby. Naturally, they were both scared and unsure of what to do. One scene showed the young man losing his cool, which didn't help matters. The girl needed the guy to stay calm and commit to see the situation through.

Finally, in an outburst of anger, the girl looked at him and said, "Somewhere inside of that pea brain of yours is a man. Access him!"[1]

Let's face it: there are lots of men out there who don't consider themselves to be leaders. You may be one of them. You may not feel mature or decisive or capable of handling the reins in a difficult situation.

On a scale of 1 to 10, how confident do you feel in your ability to lead?

1	2	3	4	5	6	7	8	9	10
Not confident at all								Fully confident	

No matter how you feel, the Scriptures are clear that God has specifically called men to lead. It started way back in the garden of Eden:

> God said, "Let us make man in our image, after our likeness. And let
> them have dominion over the fish of the sea and over the birds of
> the heavens and over the livestock and over all the earth and over
> every creeping thing that creeps on the earth." So God created
> man in his own image, in the image of God he created him; male
> and female he created them. And God blessed them. And God said
> to them, "Be fruitful and multiply and fill the earth and subdue it,
> and have dominion over the fish of the sea and over the birds of the
> heavens and over every living thing that moves on the earth."
> **GENESIS 1:26-28**

What's your initial reaction to these verses?

How do you understand the word *rule* in the context of these verses?

From the earliest moments of creation, men receive a leadership role in this world. We're stewards over creation, so we have a responsibility to care for the world around us. Of course, no individual can care for the entire world, so we all have a responsibility to ensure that God's will is carried out in our specific spheres of influence.

Several Scripture passages make it clear that men bear a larger portion of that responsibility than women. Look at 1 Corinthians 11:3, for example:

> I want you to understand that the head of every man is Christ,
> the head of a wife is her husband, and the head of Christ is God.

That doesn't mean men are more important than women, better than women, or more valuable than women. It just means men are called to carry out a specific role as leaders within their spheres of influence.

As men living in today's culture—and specifically as men seeking to follow God and do His work—we're not to be passive. We're not to shift our responsibilities onto others. The Bible teaches that we're to take the lead in our marriages, dating relationships, businesses, churches, communities, and families.

We're called to be leaders.

THE DESTRUCTIVE POWER
OF BAD LEADERS

In most sports it's pretty easy to identify when people fail to perform their roles. If an offensive lineman fails to block a hard-charging defensive end, for example, his quarterback is going to get hammered. If a power forward on an NBA team doesn't play defense, someone on the other team is going to wind up on "SportsCenter" with a spectacular dunk.

It's often more difficult to pinpoint the sources of failure in the real world. For example, who should receive the blame for the following situations?

- Your child is failing a class in school.

- Your family is forced to let the bank foreclose on the house of your dreams.

- You don't receive the promotion you applied for at work.

- Your spouse wants a divorce.

- You experience significant conflict with a family member or a former friend.

- You struggle to overcome a serious disease.

    Circle any of the previous situations you've dealt with in recent years. What emotions did you experience during those times?

    How do you typically react when you fail to do something well?

All men are called to lead, and all men have the responsibility to carry out their roles as leaders within their individual spheres of influence. But that doesn't mean all men do a good job of fulfilling those roles. Not by a long shot.

Sometimes we as men fail to lead well, and sometimes we fail even to try. Although the source of our failures isn't always obvious, the consequences of failing to lead well are clearly evident.

A BAD START

Here's a sobering thought: the first man ever created was also the first man to demonstrate poor leadership in a critical situation. We're talking about Adam, of course.

Yes, it was Eve who ate the forbidden fruit and ultimately committed the first sin, but we men need to ask an important question about that world-changing event: Where was Adam when all the bad stuff went down?

The Scriptures have the answer:

> When the woman saw that the tree was good for food, and that
> it was a delight to the eyes, and that the tree was to be desired
> to make one wise, she took of its fruit and ate, and she also
> gave some to her husband who was with her, and he ate.
> **GENESIS 3:16**

What's your initial reaction to this verse?

How does this verse reflect on Adam's role as a leader?

Let's be clear: Adam was *right there* when sin entered the world. God created him to rule in the garden—to lead, to take action when necessary. Yet he did nothing. When his wife disobeyed God's command, Adam just stood there with his hands in his pockets like a chump. (Metaphorically, of course. He didn't have pants.)

Worse, Adam took his own bite of the forbidden fruit. He failed to lead his wife by not helping her in a time of temptation, and he failed to lead by example when he did the wrong thing in a difficult situation.

Do you find it easy or difficult to take action when others make poor decisions? Explain.

Here's the thing we need to understand as men. Although Eve committed the first sin, the Bible makes it clear that God held *Adam* responsible:

> Just as sin came into the world through one man, and death
> through sin, and so death spread to all men because all sinned—
> for sin indeed was in the world before the law was given, but
> sin is not counted where there is no law. Yet death reigned from
> Adam to Moses, even over those whose sinning was not like the
> transgression of Adam, who was a type of the one who was to come.
> **ROMANS 5:12-14**

What were the consequences of Adam's failure to lead well?

How have you experienced these consequences in recent days?

Scripture is clear: the sinful nature of humankind and the broken nature of the world today can both be traced back to *one man* who sat on the sidelines during a critical situation. And it changed everything for the worse.

A GOLDEN MISTAKE

Adam isn't the only example in the Bible of a man who failed to lead well. In fact, there are dozens of such men.

Look at Aaron, for instance. He was supposed to be Moses' right-hand man while the Israelites were heading toward the promised land after the exodus from Egypt. But when Moses went to speak with God on Mount Sinai, Aaron completely failed to lead his people well.

Look at Exodus 32:1:

> When the people saw that Moses delayed to come down from the mountain, the people gathered themselves together to Aaron and said to him, "Up, make us gods who shall go before us. As for this Moses, the man who brought us up out of the land of Egypt, we do not know what has become of him."

The Israelites were afraid because they hadn't seen Moses for days and there was a huge storm surrounding the mountain. This was a chance for Aaron to take charge and steer the Israelites away from their fear and idolatry—a chance for him to stand firm and be a leader.

But he blew it. Telling the people to gather their gold, Aaron made an idol for them to worship in the shape of a calf. So instead of leading the people away from idolatry, he led them deeper into sin.

When have you been hurt or led astray because of poor leadership?

On a scale of 1 to 10, how well do you handle fear?

1	2	3	4	5	6	7	8	9	10
Not well at all									Very well

One of the more disappointing elements in this story is that Aaron wasn't even man enough to take responsibility for his failure. When Moses came charging back down the mountain and confronted him about the golden calf, Aaron blamed everyone but himself:

> Aaron said, "Let not the anger of my lord burn hot. You know the people, that they are set on evil. For they said to me, 'Make us gods who shall go before us. As for this Moses, the man who brought us up out of the land of Egypt, we do not know what has become of him.' So I said to them, 'Let any who have gold take it off.' So they gave it to me, and I threw it into the fire, and out came this calf."
> **EXODUS 32:22-24**

"It's the people's fault. They're set on evil, and they brought me all this gold. All I did was throw it in the fire, and out came a calf—like magic!"

How was Aaron's failure similar to Adam's?

Look at Genesis 3:8-13. How was Aaron's response to his failure similar to Adam's response in the garden of Eden?

There are many more examples of failed leaders in the Bible. Moses himself made several mistakes, as did guys like Samson, Saul, David, Peter, and so on. All of them caused damage because of their failures and mistakes, just as we cause damage whenever we miss the mark as leaders today.

Fortunately, the Bible tells us one Man always did the right thing as a leader. We'll talk more about Him and what He can teach us as we finish up this week's study.

LEADERSHIP AND YOU

MATT'S STORY

A while back I was standing around talking with a group of people at a backyard event associated with my church when I noticed a little boy hanging around as if he didn't have anything to do. He was about 10 years old, the same age as my daughter, so I walked over to have a friendly chat.

I started by asking where his dad was. "On a business trip," the boy said. "He's going to be gone for a couple of weeks."

"Oh. Do you miss your dad when he's gone like that?"

"Nah, not really."

I was shocked. "How come?" I asked.

"Well, he's never around even when he's home," the boy said. "When he is, he's always in his office working. I see him only a few minutes each day. Honestly, he doesn't pay much attention to us."

In less than seven seconds that boy spoke a mouthful. In fact, it broke my heart. I was expecting to hear the opposite—that he missed his dad greatly. I certainly hope if I were gone on business and somebody asked my kids if they missed me, they'd say, "Absolutely."

Now I don't know this boy's father, and I don't know the specific circumstances of this family's life. Maybe the father doesn't have a choice to live differently than he's doing right now. Or maybe the boy was just having a bad day and venting about his father's being gone.

Either way, though, the situation wasn't working for that family. Something was wrong, damage was being done, and it all pointed to a failure in leadership on one level or another.

What are the primary ways you serve as a leader within your spheres of influence?

When have you failed to lead well in those areas?

What consequences have you seen as a result of those failures?

FOLLOWING THE LEADER

We started this study by exploring the need for modern men to redefine *success*—to move away from our culture's definition of a good life and instead concentrate on trusting God and serving Him. That's the real win.

We've been talking this week about leadership. All men are created to lead within their specific spheres of influence, and in doing so, we help others experience the real win as well. When we fulfill our roles as leaders, we guide our family, friends, neighbors, and coworkers to experience authentic success for themselves.

Unfortunately, we don't always lead the right way. We mess up sometimes, and our failures often cause damage to the people we care most about—as in the story of the little boy and his father.

Basically, we have two conflicting ideas: (1) men are called to lead, but (2) men often fail in their attempts to lead well. How can we reconcile those two statements? How can men fulfill our roles as leaders in spite of our failures?

What's your initial reaction to the previous questions?

How does our culture typically react to the failures of those who lead?

The first thing to keep in mind is that men aren't called to perfection. Yes, we need to do our best in all situations, but James 3:2 makes it clear that "we all stumble in many ways." That certainly includes men who serve as leaders. Romans 3:23 reminds us that we "all have sinned and fall short of the glory of God."

If we ignore these realities, we only makes things worse because we end up refusing to admit our failures, as Adam and Aaron did.

Do you feel pressure to avoid mistakes as a man or as a follower of God? Explain.

On a scale of 1 to 10, how difficult is it for you to admit when you've messed up?

1	2	3	4	5	6	7	8	9	10
Not difficult									Very difficult

The solution to dealing with your failures isn't simply to try harder. You've probably been down that road, haven't you? You make a mistake, and you think, *Next time I'll do better. Next time I'll work harder or pray more, and things will be different.* But how'd that work out for you?

> **When have you tried to avoid mistakes by working harder?**
> **What happened?**

Again, we're broken. We're sinful. We don't have the capacity to fix what's wrong with us, so we'll continue to fail no matter how hard we try to do things better next time. So how can we function well as men whom God has called to lead?

The answer is to turn to Jesus and throw ourselves into pursuing Him—to serve Him because we trust Him and we know that *He* will lead us in the right direction even when we have no idea what to do or where to go.

In other words, we've talked about redefining success, but we also need to redefine leadership. Only to the extent that we follow Jesus will we be able to lead those whom God has entrusted to us. The apostle Paul gave us a clear picture of this reality in this passage from the Book of Romans:

> If, because of one man's trespass, death reigned through that one
> man, much more will those who receive the abundance of grace and
> the free gift of righteousness reign in life through the one man Jesus
> Christ. Therefore, as one trespass led to condemnation for all men,
> so one act of righteousness leads to justification and life for all men.
> **ROMANS 5:17-18**

Do you see the logic here? Even though sin entered the world through the failures of the first man, Adam, the restoring work of Jesus Christ trumps all Adam ever did. Because Jesus perfectly fulfilled His role as a leader, we don't have to be perfect ourselves. Rather, we have "the abundance of grace and the free gift of righteousness" (v. 17). That's why Paul could say, "Follow my example, as I follow the example of Christ" (1 Cor. 11:1, NIV).

Jesus is the only Man who ever lived perfectly—the only Leader who ever fulfilled His role without any mistakes. He died on the cross, was raised in power, and now lives in us and gives us the ability to walk boldly through life and lead more and more like Him each day.

Therefore, trusting Jesus is the only hope we have to lead well as men. Serving Jesus is the only way we can fulfill our roles and benefit those we care about.

How does your relationship with Jesus affect your leadership in the following areas?

At home:

At work:

In your neighborhood:

In your church:

As a man, you're called to lead. And as a human being, you're going to stumble at times in your efforts to obey that call. Thankfully, the way for us to deal with our failures as men and as leaders is to follow Jesus. That means going where He wants us to go and doing what He wants us to do—seeking, obeying, and depending on Him rather than trying to figure everything out ourselves. That's how we live up to the call God has placed on our lives as men.

1. "Wheels," episode 9 of "Glee," originally aired November 11, 2009.

IDOLATRY

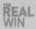

WELCOME BACK
TO THIS GROUP DISCUSSION OF *THE REAL WIN.*

The previous session's application activity challenged you to submit yourself to Jesus' leadership by studying His Word and praying each day. If you're comfortable, talk about your recent experiences with those disciplines.

Describe what you liked best about the study material in week 2. What questions do you have?

ACTIVITY. Spend several minutes as a group answering the question, What do people desire most in today's society? Start by going through newspapers, magazines, and/or catalogs and cutting out pictures of people, places, and things that represent the strongest desires of people in our culture. After you've cut out several pictures, use the following questions to guide your discussion.

- How do the pictures you've cut out represent the desires present in today's culture?

- What are some common elements among the pictures you've chosen as a group?

- What makes our desires and cravings either appropriate or inappropriate?

To prepare to watch the DVD segment, read aloud the following verses.

> I have seen the business that God has given to the children of
> man to be busy with. He has made everything beautiful in its time.
> Also, he has put eternity into man's heart, yet so that he cannot
> find out what God has done from the beginning to the end.
> **ECCLESIASTES 3:10-11**

WATCH DVD session 3.

DISCUSS the DVD segment with your group, using the following questions.

What did you like best about the visual elements in the DVD segment?

What did you like best about the discussion between Colt and Matt? Why?

How would you define the sin of idolatry in today's world?

When have your cravings and desires led you to cross the line into idolatry?

What's your reaction to Matt's four classifications of idols: power, comfort, approval, and control?

Colt shared that he most often struggles with the idol of power. What idol(s) have you dealt with in recent months?

How can we as a group work to support and encourage one another in the battle against idolatry?

APPLICATION. One key to resisting idolatry is to remain focused on worshiping God above all other people, places, or things. Identify something you can carry around with you this week as a reminder to continually worship God. Write down this week's Scripture-memory verse and keep it in your pocket, for example, or tape it to the dashboard of your car. Whatever you choose, commit to concentrate on intentionally worshiping God each day this week.

THIS WEEK'S SCRIPTURE MEMORY. Psalm 37:4:

> Delight yourself in the LORD,
> and he will give you the desires of your heart.

ASSIGNMENT. Read week 3 and complete the activities before the next group experience.

Spotting the **Hook**

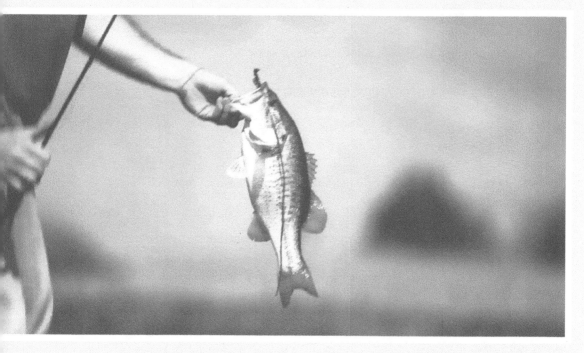

The sport of fishing has become increasingly complicated in recent years. Improvements in technology mean you can spend thousands of dollars on sophisticated boats, baits, rods, depth finders, and more. You can study maps, charts, and seasons and pour hours into determining where the biggest fish will be and what's required to catch them.

But when you get down to it, the basic idea of fishing has remained unchanged for thousands of years: you catch a fish by offering it something that looks enticing but ultimately leaves the fish dangling on the end of your line.

Of course, the key element from a fisherman's perspective is the hook. That's what enables you to snare the fish and make it yours once it decides to take the bait.

This week we're going to look at the concept of idolatry. That's not a word we use often today, even in the church, and it's a concept we don't usually apply to our modern lives. But we should.

Whether or not we recognize it, idolatry is present in the heart of every person. It's a deep-seated sin that diverts us from God's plan for authentic success to pursue goals and achievements that are ultimately worthless.

As we'll see in the pages to come, these false pursuits cause an incredible amount of damage to our souls. They bring wave after wave of pain and disappointment in our lives. Because idolatry always comes with a hook.

DEFINING *IDOLATRY*

MATT'S STORY

As of the writing of this study, Austin Stone Community Church is 10 years old. Those 10 years have gone by so fast! Seriously, I can't believe a decade ago I was just starting this good work.

But here's my confession. My daughter, Annie, was born right around the time we planted the church, and I have almost no memories of my sweet little girl's first two years of life. That fact devastates me. I was so involved with planting my church, so consumed with making sure everything ran smoothly, so absorbed in pursuing my goal and creating a successful ministry, that I missed out on an important part of my princess's young life.

My wife is a down-to-earth Southern beauty who doesn't pull punches, so she'll tell you that I flat-out ignored my family for several years. It's not that I didn't love my wife and kids; it's just that I was consumed with my job. The church had become a mistress to me. I had a love affair with my career, and it stole my rightful allegiances.

Thankfully, I've reconciled things with my family in recent years, and I've brought my life more into balance. But I think my story is a common one, which is why I need to ask the question: Men, why do things like this happen? Why, in our quest for success and achievement, do we so easily lose sight of what's most important?

For example:

- Why do some men drive themselves so hard at work that they lose the hearts of their wives and kids?

- Why do some men—even men who demonstrate integrity in most situations— bend ethical standards to succeed in business?

- Why do so many men keep looking at pornography, even when they don't want to, in an attempt to find satisfaction?

- Why do young men break their standards and take unchangeable actions simply because they want the approval of their peers?

- Why do so many men turn to anger and outrage when they feel disrespected or unloved?

I think idolatry is the often-overlooked answer to many of these questions. It's the root that drives us toward unrealistic and unfulfilling definitions of *success*. That was true of me, and I believe it's true of many other men today. Maybe it's even true of you.

Let's explore that concept together and find out.

Which of the previous situations have you experienced in recent years?

What steps have you taken to avoid or resolve those issues?

What ideas or images come to mind when you hear the word *idolatry*?

UNDERSTANDING IDOLATRY

Most of us understand from history and archaeology that in ancient cultures, people worshiped physical idols. They created a statue or carving out of wood, metal, or stone, and then they bowed down in front of their creation and worshiped it as a god. They even went so far as to slaughter animals or their own children and burn them as offerings to these idols.

That sounds kind of silly, right? For those of us living in a modern, Western culture, the idea of worshiping something we built with our own hands seems ridiculous. We understand what the prophet Isaiah was getting at when he wrote these words about an idolater:

He cuts down cedars. ... Then it becomes fuel for a man. He takes
a part of it and warms himself; he kindles a fire and bakes bread.
Also he makes a god and worships it; he makes it an idol and
falls down before it. Half of it he burns in the fire. Over the half
he eats meat; he roasts it and is satisfied. Also he warms himself
and says, "Aha, I am warm, I have seen the fire!" And the rest of
it he makes into a god, his idol, and falls down to it and worships
it. He prays to it and says, "Deliver me, for you are my god!"
ISAIAH 44:14-17

How would you summarize Isaiah's main point in these verses?

What motivates people to create their own paths to God, forgiveness, and salvation?

Basically, most of us think of idols and idolatry as ideas that are kind of out there—concepts that don't have any application to our everyday lives. Unfortunately, we're wrong. That's because the definition of *idolatry* isn't limited to worshiping a physical idol.

Rather, a more comprehensive definition of *idolatry* is *pursuing anything more than you pursue God*. It's worshiping or desiring anything more than you worship and desire God.

What emotions do you experience when you read this definition of *idolatry*? Why?

Idolatry is a major problem in today's society. It's a major problem even within the church and among those of us attempting to follow Jesus. Why? Because it's so easy for us to drift into pursuing our own definitions of *success* or our own desires more than we pursue God and what He's planned for us.

And when that happens—when idolatry takes up residence in our hearts—it becomes more destructive to our souls than we can possibly imagine. If you don't believe us about that, look back at what King Solomon had to say in the Book of Ecclesiastes.

Solomon was the wisest and most successful man of his day. He had everything: money, power, fame, and respect. He ate the best foods, drank the best wine, wore the best clothes, and listened to the best music. He even had a harem filled with hundreds of the most beautiful women in the land. He literally became the most powerful man in the world, and he was denied nothing he desired.

Here's what he ultimately concluded about the whole situation:

> I the Preacher have been king over Israel in Jerusalem. And I applied
> my heart to seek and to search out by wisdom all that is done
> under heaven. It is an unhappy business that God has given to the
> children of man to be busy with. I have seen everything that is done
> under the sun, and behold, all is vanity and a striving after wind.
> **ECCLESIASTES 1:12-14**

What's your initial reaction to these verses? Why?

Do you agree or disagree with Solomon's conclusion? Explain.

You'd think a man who had it all would be supremely happy—that he'd feel content, satisfied, and respected, as if he had it all together. But in the end Solomon determined that all he had accumulated and experienced was worth nothing and meaningless.

How have you seen Solomon's experience play out in the life of someone you know?

How have you experienced a sense of futility in your pursuits?

Later in Ecclesiastes Solomon explained why none of his pursuits and achievements could bring satisfaction:

> I have seen the business that God has given to the children of
> man to be busy with. He has made everything beautiful in its time.
> Also, he has put eternity into man's heart, yet so that he cannot
> find out what God has done from the beginning to the end.
> **ECCLESIASTES 3:10-11**

That word *eternity* is the key to this verse. Solomon realized that God has placed in every human heart a longing for something that really matters—something that's eternal. And who or what is eternal? God.

Whether or not we realize it, all of us are fueled by a built-in longing for eternity—for God. And for that reason we won't be satisfied by anything that isn't eternal. We can't find fulfillment or purpose in anything that isn't God Himself.

That's why idolatry is so destructive. It pushes us to pursue noneternal things more than we pursue God. It drives us to spend our lives striving for people, possessions, or accomplishments that can't ever fill the deepest needs of our hearts.

FOUR TYPES OF IDOLS

Take a moment to think about a shovel—just an ordinary shovel like the one you keep in your toolshed or garage. Get a picture of that shovel in your mind. You can even make a sketch in the margin.

The thing about a shovel is that it has only one purpose. Other tools—hammers, screwdrivers, knives—can do several different kinds of jobs. But a shovel is good for only one thing: digging. It's specifically designed to cut through a bunch of dirt, gravel, or sand and then toss it aside to make space for something else.

Now why are we making a big deal about shovels? Because we need you to do some digging over these next few pages. Earlier we said the reason many of us continually struggle with idolatry is that we spend our lives trying to find things to meet a need in our hearts that only God can truly satisfy. We pursue those goals, desires, or achievements more than we pursue God, and it never works.

That's one reason so many men feel dissatisfied with their marriage; they're looking to their wife to meet a need she doesn't have the ability to meet. That's also why so many single men struggle with contentment in the midst of their singleness; they're looking for a human relationship to meet a need it wasn't designed to meet. That's why so many men feel discontented with their jobs, their houses, their cars, or their bodies; they're trying to use created things to fulfill a desire that can be fulfilled only by the Creator.

If you're serious about the real win, you need to grab a shovel and go to work on your heart. You've got to dig through the surface layers of your spirituality and your idea of what you're supposed to think. You've got to expose the problems under-neath—the idols you're pursuing instead of God. Only when those idols are laid bare can you confess them to God and move forward toward authentic success.

> When have you recently examined what's going on in your heart and mind—a motive, a concern, or a desire? What did you discover?

Let's take a look at four major types of idols pursued by men like us.

THE IDOL OF POWER

The desire for power is huge in the hearts of men. That's not necessarily a bad thing. After all, power is the capability to accomplish something important and influence others positively. But power becomes an idol when we worship it—when we pursue it as something above God and more valuable than God.

To bow before the idol of power is to say, "I have worth when I have influence, recognition, and fame. I feel important when I can cause people to do what I want, when I want, exactly as I want it done." The idol of power, then, tempts us to usurp God's place as Creator and King within our spheres of influence.

How does our culture view the concept of power?

What does it look like for someone to have power in today's world?

Is it possible you may uncover the idol of power when you look into the deepest layers of your heart? Circle *yes* or *no* beside each statement below to start digging.

You have a strong desire for authority over people. You *need* to be in charge.	YES	NO
Humiliation is one of your greatest fears.	YES	NO
You're quick to feel slighted or disrespected by others.	YES	NO
You strongly dislike it when you tell people to do something and they do something else.	YES	NO
You struggle with giving credit to others for their accomplishments, and you quickly become angry or jealous when you don't receive credit for yours.	YES	NO

As Christians, we have access to the power of God's Spirit indwelling us and enabling us to accomplish impossible things. But too often we settle for the fast-food version of power. We're not interested in working for the power that comes only from humbling ourselves in prayer and asking God to move, so we grasp and grab for worldy power instead.

Do you struggle with pursuing power as an idol? Explain.

THE IDOL OF CONTROL

To control something means to regulate or restrain it. In the right situation, for someone who has the right authority, control can be a good or even necessary thing. But many people feel a need to know exactly what's happening in every area of their lives. They feel a drive to manipulate their circumstances in order to achieve the exact outcomes they're looking for. This leads to idolatry.

When people worship the idol of control, they say, "I'm content and at peace only if I'm able to get mastery over a certain area of my life" or "I'm happy only when things are occurring according to my plans and desires." So the idol of control tempts us to usurp God's place as Lord and Master, both in our own lives and in the lives of those we want to manage.

How does our culture view the practice of control?

What emotions do you experience when others attempt to control you? Why?

The sad thing is that we have a Heavenly Father who's in control of all things, yet we refuse to let go of the reins because we want to know the future rather than the One who holds the future in His hands.

Use the following chart to explore whether control may be an idol in your life.

You quickly experience fear, anger, or anxiety when circumstances deviate from your plans.	YES	NO
You easily become frustrated or stressed when people are late or don't follow your schedule.	YES	NO
Chaos and confusion are among your greatest fears.	YES	NO
You feel rigidly attached to budgets and other plans for allocating resources.	YES	NO
You have specific, detailed plans for many areas of your life.	YES	NO

Do you struggle with pursuing control as an idol? Explain.

THE IDOL OF COMFORT

Comfort is the feeling of being soothed, consoled, relieved, or reassured. Let's be honest: we all need comfort at different times in our lives. But some people go after comfort as if it were a divine right. They demand large portions of ease and even luxury in their lives. These people say, "I'm happy only when I have a high standard of living" or "The best days are when I find a variety of ways to push my pleasure buttons." In this way the idol of comfort tempts us to usurp God's role as Provider and Sustainer.

How does our culture respond to the innate desire for comfort and pleasure?

In what situations do you feel most comfortable and at ease?

Use the following chart to explore whether your pursuit of comfort may be an idol in your life.

When confronted by choices and opportunities, you almost always take the easiest road.	YES	NO
You expend a lot of effort to avoid stress and difficult situations.	YES	NO
You deal with trials by turning to food, pornography, entertainment, or other forms of pleasure.	YES	NO
Poverty and abstinence are among your greatest fears.	YES	NO
You block off large portions of each day for "me time."	YES	NO

So often we settle for a counterfeit form of comfort. We want to make peace with our sin instead of warring against it and killing it. We settle for the easy way out, and we retreat from the battleground even though God offers us a victory party once we've taken the enemy ground.

Do you struggle with pursuing comfort as an idol? Explain.

THE IDOL OF APPROVAL

Approval is what occurs when people praise you, judge you favorably, agree with you, or consistently commend you for a job well done. And who doesn't want approval? We all need to be affirmed to one degree or another. But the desire for others' approval can quickly get out of hand.

When approval is your idol, you're not content or at peace unless you're loved or accepted by most of the people around you. People who bow before the idol of approval say, "I love being loved. I need to be needed. Life is unbearable when people don't know how good I really am." Therefore, the idol of approval tempts us to use others to usurp God's role as Father.

How does our culture view the concept of approval?

Who are the main sources of the approval you receive day in and day out?

Use the following chart to explore whether approval is an idol in your life.

Your day is ruined if you receive a negative comment or criticism.	YES	NO
You strongly consider what others will think of you when you're faced with important decisions.	YES	NO
You feel compelled to check how many people are following you or responding to you through social media.	YES	NO
Being forgotten or left out is one of your greatest fears.	YES	NO
You tend to smother those with whom you have a close relationship.	YES	NO

Our desires for power, control, comfort, and approval aren't wrong in and of themselves. All of these desires are proper desires if placed within the context of eternity and if submitted to the lordship of Christ. The problem comes when we try to short-circuit eternity and seek a counterfeit version of the desires God has placed in our hearts.

Idolatry is real, and we all experience it to one degree or another. Idolatry is damaging, and we'll continue to be unsatisfied as long as we pursue trivial things instead of our eternal God.

So quit pursuing your idols. Run to Jesus instead, because that's where your real win will be.

IDOLATRY AND YOU

COLT'S STORY

I know I've struggled with idolatry in the past, and I'm sure I'll continue feeling the urge to run away from God and pursue things that are ultimately unimportant. For me, that's typically involved the idol of power.

For example, toward the end of my college football career, there was a lot of talk saying that I was in a good position to be drafted, maybe even in the first round. That's certainly something I was striving for. But after my injury in the national-championship game, there were concerns about my shoulder holding up over the long haul. So instead of achieving my goal of being a first-round pick, I ended up getting drafted in the third round.

Now being a third-round pick in the NFL is certainly a great opportunity, and I really don't mean to complain, but it wasn't all I was hoping for. There are lots of reasons my situation grated on me. Honestly, one of them was financial. The dif-ference between my salary as a third-round pick and that of a first-round pick was literally millions of dollars. More importantly, there were 84 guys drafted ahead of me by NFL teams. That hurt my pride.

Again, I was struggling with the pursuit of power—with my desire to be the best. The draft results made it clear that I wasn't the man anymore; I wasn't on top, even on my own team. Also, I felt a little disappointed in God. I felt that this was another situation in which I was set up to receive a blessing, but I was ultimately let down.

Things didn't get any easier my first year with the Cleveland Browns. My head coach, Eric Mangini, told me that he'd never had a rookie quarterback play for him, so he wanted my first year to be a watching-and-learning year. Our starting quarterback was the talented Jake Delhomme, and his backup was Seneca Wallace, a nine-year veteran of the NFL. That meant I wasn't going to play.

For a guy who'd been the starting quarterback at the University of Texas, that was a major disappointment. I hadn't missed a start in four years, but now I'd be watching our games from the sidelines.

Thankfully, God didn't waste my feelings of discontentment. As I poured myself into training each day, I began to recognize that idolatry was ultimately the source of my disappointment. I realized that all men turn to different things in an effort to feel fulfilled, valued, satisfied, or relieved, and I was trying to pursue power.

I thought if I could just get on top and be the best, everything would get better. But through prayer, studying the Scripture, and conversations with Matt, I finally understood that only God could satisfy the strongest desires inside me. Unless I turned to Him, I'd continue to feel disappointed, no matter how successful my career became.

I love being an NFL quarterback. I couldn't be happier about getting to practice and train and go hard with my teammates every day. But if my heart had been set only on winning games, winning awards, and being the best, I'd have been on the verge of despair more than once in recent years.

Achievement is still important to me, of course. I want to win. I get up every day and work my tail off to become a successful quarterback, and I hope something great is going to happen as I continue in my career. I'm shooting to lead my team well, be the best player I can be, and take my team to the Super Bowl someday.

But ultimately, my heart is set on something greater than all of those goals. I've realized that being a great quarterback isn't my only purpose in life; it's not even my primary purpose. Instead, my purpose is serving God and trusting Him. That involves serving my wife, leading my family, loving my teammates and coaches, reaching out to my community, and being the best follower of Christ I can be.

What are some goals in your life that you haven't yet achieved?

What will happen if you never achieve those goals? How will it affect you?

How would you describe the primary purpose of your life in recent years?

CONFRONTING IDOLATRY

When you give advice to people or explain the rules in a certain situation, don't you start with the most important stuff first? That makes the most sense. And that's why we need to pay attention to God's first statement in the Ten Commandments:

> You shall have no other gods before me. You shall not make for
> yourself a carved image, or any likeness of anything that is in
> heaven above, or that is in the earth beneath, or that is in the water
> under the earth. You shall not bow down to them or serve them.
> **EXODUS 20:3-5**

Think about that for a moment: God commanded His people to fight against idolatry *before* He commanded them not to murder one another. God talked about idolatry before He talked about adultery, stealing, or lying.

If you're still feeling that idolatry isn't that big a deal in your life, then this needs to be the moment you give in and get with the program. Idolatry is a huge deal to God. Idolatry is present in our lives, and it's more destructive than we can imagine.

In what ways have you seen idolatry promoted by today's culture?

In what areas do you struggle with idolatry today?

We've talked about the four broad categories of idols that men often struggle with: power, control, comfort, and approval. So how do we deal with these idols? How do we confront them and actively seek to stop pursuing them?

The first step is to realize that we don't have to do this on our own. In fact, we *can't* do this on our own. God doesn't want us to spend our lives pursuing things that can't satisfy us, and He's willing to help. In addition, He's promised to help.

Look at Philippians 1:6:

> I am sure of this, that he who began a good work in you
> will bring it to completion at the day of Jesus Christ.

Scripture promises that God has been working in your life every day since you became a Christian to help you become more like Jesus, and He will continue working until the day you see Him face-to-face. You're not in this alone, and you don't have to rely on your own strength and willpower to step away from idols.

How have you changed since you decided to follow God?

What has God brought about that you couldn't have achieved on your own?

There are two ways God goes about highlighting and removing idols from our hearts.

1. Sometimes God prevents us from experiencing the things we want so badly. In other words, He keeps us from achieving goals that are driven by idolatry. So God may withhold something you desire until you get to the place where you truly pursue Him above anything else.

2. Sometimes God actually lets you have the thing you're longing for in order to prove that it can't meet your heart's desire. He gives you what you want and then allows you to feel the disappointment and despair that come with realizing that you're still not satisfied. That's what happened with Solomon, of course. He had everything, and it drove him to realize that only God could satisfy his deepest desires.

Think back to the goals in life you haven't yet achieved. Are your efforts to achieve those goals driving you toward God or away from Him? Explain.

When have you recently achieved a goal or fulfilled a desire that left you feeling disappointed?

Does all this mean we're supposed to sit back passively and wait for God to do the work of removing our idols? No, that's not what we're saying at all.

Our job is to pursue God with everything we have—to pour our energy and resources into trusting Him and serving Him every hour of every day. That's authentic success, and that's our best weapon in the fight against idolatry.

So we can pursue God and fight against idolatry by studying God's Word every day—by submitting to the truths He's communicated in the Bible. We can do it by spending time in prayer throughout the day, not just when we need something or want something from God but simply to talk with Him about our dreams, fears, failures, and hopes. We can fight idolatry by practicing other spiritual disciplines such as fasting, memorizing Scripture, praising God, and more.

We can also pursue God and battle idolatry by obeying God's commands. For example, we can find practical ways to love our neighbors as ourselves (see Matt. 22:39) or to care for widows and orphans (see Jas. 1:27). Obedience demonstrates our submission to God's priorities for our lives.

Let's finish with a verse from that can help us keep in mind our primary goal of pursuing God:

> Delight yourself in the LORD,
> and he will give you the desires of your heart.
> **PSALM 37:4**

What's your initial reaction to this verse? Why?

It's easy to give that verse a quick glance and think, *Wow, if I delight myself in the Lord, He will give me anything I want.* But that's not what the verse actually says.

Instead, the psalmist was helping us see that if and when we delight in the Lord instead of all the other junk we pursue—if we allow God to satisfy us instead of seeking satisfaction in counterfeit desires—then He will give us what our hearts long for most. He will give us what we truly desire, because what we truly desire will be God.

And that's the real win.

WORK

WELCOME BACK
TO THIS GROUP DISCUSSION OF *THE REAL WIN.*

The previous session's application activity challenged you to focus on the worship of God above everything else. If you're comfortable, talk about your ability to focus on God throughout the week and any encounters with Him you'd like to share.

Describe what you liked best about the study material in week 3. What questions do you have?

ACTIVITY. As a group, explore the following list of activities. Then give examples of how each activity could be viewed as both work and fun. For instance, if the activity were reading a book, you could give reading for relaxation as an example of fun. And you could give reading a technical manual as an example of work.

- Tying a rope

- Building a fire

- Digging a hole

- Using a brush

What ideas or images come to mind when you hear the word *work*?

To prepare to watch the DVD segment, read aloud the following verses.

> The LORD God formed the man of dust from the ground and breathed
> into his nostrils the breath of life, and the man became a living
> creature. And the LORD God planted a garden in Eden, in the east,
> and there he put the man whom he had formed. The LORD God took
> the man and put him in the garden of Eden to work it and keep it.
> **GENESIS 2:7-8,15**

WATCH DVD session 4.

DISCUSS the DVD segment with your group, using the following questions.

What did you like best about the visual elements in the DVD segment?

What did you like best about the discussion between Colt and Matt? Why?

Who among your friends and family has modeled a strong work ethic for you?

What do you like best about the work you currently do?

What do you like least about the work you currently do?

Respond to Colt's statement: "Whatever you are doing, whatever you've been called to do, whether you like it or not, your call is to work for the Lord."

How can you bring glory to God through your work this week?

APPLICATION. You already have a good idea of the types of work you dislike most, and you likely already know when you'll have to engage in those types of work this week. Therefore, seek to use those times to your advantage by intentionally dedicating your least favorite types of work to God as an effort to glorify Him. Pray to God before you start your least favories activites and continue praying while you're working that He will be glorified and will make your efforts count.

THIS WEEK'S SCRIPTURE MEMORY. Colossians 3:23-24:

> Whatever you do, work heartily, as for the Lord and not for men,
> knowing that from the Lord you will receive the inheritance
> as your reward. You are serving the Lord Christ.

ASSIGNMENT. Read week 4 and complete the activities before the next group experience.

Work or **Fun**?

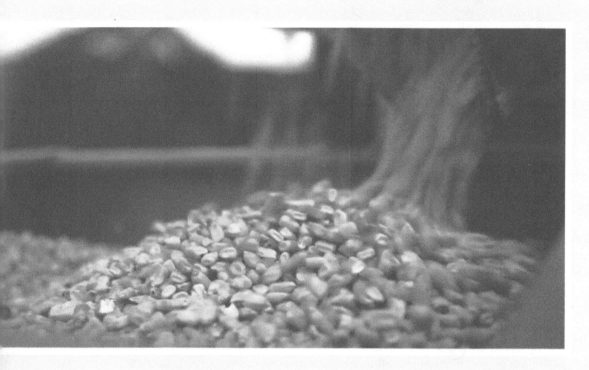

There are lots of ways to have fun in the world today, and many of them require very little effort on our part. For example, you can pick up a TV remote or a video-game controller and entertain yourself almost immediately. Or you can snatch up a football, walk into the backyard with a buddy, and play a little catch without any preparation.

When it comes to outdoor activities like hunting and fishing, however, most people have to put in a good amount of work before they can have a little fun.

For fishing it's important to find the right bait to match the fish you're trying to catch. You need to maintain your equipment and prepare your rod before going out. You need to identify the right time to fish, hitch up your boat to your trailer, and usually drive awhile to find the perfect spot. It takes work to fish.

It takes even more work to hunt. Most hunters spend hours and hours maintaining their property by filling feeders, building tree stands or blinds, and clearing out brush and branches to keep a good line of site. You have to be disciplined in maintaining your equipment. You typically have to wake up before the sun in order to hunt, and you probably have to stay up late the night before to keep things scented properly and arrange everything just right. It takes work.

So here's a question. What's the difference between the work we put in before having fun and the work we do in our jobs every day? Why does one kind of work seem natural and positive, while the other kind of work so often drives us crazy?

We'll address that question and a lot of others this week as we explore this idea of work and how it helps us achieve the real win in our lives.

WORK: A QUICK HISTORY

MATT'S STORY

A while back I read a fascinating book called *Open*. It's the autobiography of Andre Agassi, one of the most recognizable tennis stars ever to play the game.

I knew from my friendship with Colt that being a professional athlete doesn't automatically mean you have an easy, carefree life. But I'd always assumed that people who dedicated their lives to a specific sport did so because they enjoyed that sport so much—especially someone like Andre Agassi, who spent more than 20 years as a pro. That makes sense, right?

But look at what Agassi had to say about his job as a tennis player:

> My name is Andre Agassi. My wife's name is Stefanie Graf. We have two children, a son and a daughter, five and three. We live in Las Vegas, Nevada, but currently reside in a suite at the Four Seasons Hotel in New York City, because I'm playing in the 2006 U.S. Open. My last U.S. Open. In fact my last tournament ever. I play tennis for a living, even though I hate tennis, hate it with a dark and secret passion, and always have.[1]

Isn't that incredible? I picked up the book in an airport bookstore and skimmed the first page until I saw that last sentence. I was hooked! I had to read more.

Truth be told, that's how many men feel about their work. Maybe even you. In fact, could this be your testimony?

> Hi, my name is _____, and I do XYZ for a living, even though I hate XYZ, hate it with a dark and secret passion, and always have.

I'm fortunate enough to be in a position where I really enjoy what I do for a living, but I fully understand that many men literally *hate* their jobs. They hate hearing the alarm clock go off every morning. They hate fighting traffic. They hate dealing with caustic coworkers or ungrateful customers. They hate leaving their families for 8, 9, 10, or even 12 hours a day.

And even those of us who don't hate our jobs often struggle to find any meaningful purpose in what we do. We sometimes wonder, *What's this all about? Does my work have any eternal significance? Am I wasting my life with what I do?*

Here's the good news: we don't have to feel like Andre Agassi. We don't have to ask those tough questions about the work we do day after day. Instead, we can find joy and purpose in our work, even when our jobs aren't fun or inspiring.

That's because God invites us to follow Him wholeheartedly in every area of our lives, including the jobs we do to make a living.

Record three things you like most about the work you currently do.
1.

2.

3.

Record three things you dislike most about your current work.
1.

2.

3.

How does work help you experience God?

GOOD WORK TURNED BAD
The Bible has a lot to say about the subject of work, so we'll explore several Scripture passages over the next several pages. The best place to get started is with our friend Adam, the first man ever to land a job:

> The LORD God formed the man of dust from the ground and breathed
> into his nostrils the breath of life, and the man became a living
> creature. And the LORD God planted a garden in Eden, in the east,
> and there he put the man whom he had formed. The LORD God took
> the man and put him in the garden of Eden to work it and keep it.
> **GENESIS 2:7-8,15**

What do these verses teach about work?

Notice that Adam (and later Eve) was placed in the garden of Eden with a specific purpose: to work. He was to cultivate the plant life, and he also had dominion over the animals, even to the point of giving a name to every living thing he encountered (see Gen. 2:19).

Also notice that Adam's call to work came in Genesis 2. Why is that important? Because sin didn't enter the world until Genesis 3, a chapter later. In other words, God commanded Adam to get to work while everything was still unblemished and perfect. Work was part of God's plan from the beginning.

Don't miss the significance of that fact. So often we think of work as something evil or as punishment for Adam's sin. We think before the fall Adam and Eve were just lying around all day, eating fruit and being naked. But the truth is that they were working, even at the beginning. And it was a good thing.

Work isn't evil. Work isn't punishment for sin or a by-product of the fall. No, work is ordained by God.

What's your reaction to the previous statements?

Unfortunately, that wasn't the end of the story. The fall happened. Sin entered the world and corrupted everything, including work. Here's what God said to Adam in Genesis 3:

Because you have listened to the voice of your wife
and have eaten of the tree
of which I commanded you, "You shall not eat of it,"
cursed is the ground because of you;
in pain you shall eat of it all the days of your life;
thorns and thistles it shall bring forth for you;
and you shall eat the plants of the field.
By the sweat of your face
you shall eat bread,
till you return to the ground,
for out of it you were taken;
for you are dust,
and to dust you shall return.
GENESIS 3:17-19

What do these verses teach about work?

List the ways sin corrupted work, according to these verses.

How have you experienced these consequences in your own work?

Do you see how drastic the change was for work before and after the fall? This is why, thousands of years later, one of the best tennis players of all time—a career athlete who made hundreds of millions of dollars playing tennis and inspiring thousands of fans the world over—would describe his work so negatively: "I play tennis for a living, even though I hate tennis, hate it with a dark and secret passion, and always have."

Fortunately, we don't have to end there.

UNDERSTANDING OUR WORK

We're taking a deeper look at the subject of work this week, a subject we're all intimately familiar with. So far we've seen that work was always part of God's plan and originally a good thing, but it was corrupted by sin along with everything else in this world. Consequently, work has become a source of drudgery, frustration, and pain for many people in the world today.

That brings us to these words from Solomon:

> I made great works. I built houses and planted vineyards for myself.
> I made myself gardens and parks, and planted in them all kinds
> of fruit trees. I made myself pools from which to water the forest
> of growing trees. I bought male and female slaves, and had slaves
> who were born in my house. I had also great possessions of herds
> and flocks, more than any who had been before me in Jerusalem.
> **Then I considered all that my hands had done and the toil I had
> expended in doing it, and behold, all was vanity and a striving
> after wind, and there was nothing to be gained under the sun.**
> **ECCLESIASTES 2:4-7,11, EMPHASIS ADDED**

What's your initial reaction to these verses?

Record three recent accomplishments at work that you're most proud of.
1.

2.

3.

We emphasized Ecclesiastes 2:11 because it's something you need to wrestle with. Solomon, one of the wisest people who ever lived, achieved more through his work than most of us could even dream of accomplishing. And yet he referred to it all as vanity—like chasing the wind.

So this is what Scripture teaches about work in a world that's still corrupted by sin: in your most financially profitable year, during your greatest quarter of productivity, whenever you're most applauded and promoted and find the most satisfaction in your work, if you haven't discovered a God-ordained purpose for your job, you're laboring in vain!

How do your experiences with work compare to the previous statement?

Fortunately, there's good news for us on this subject of work: the news of reconciliation.

RECONCILING OUR WORK

If you're not familiar with that term, *reconciliation* refers to restoring something that was broken or connecting two or more things that were separated in the past. It's a term that implies fixing something that was once broken.

What ideas or images come to mind when you hear the word *reconciliation?*

Christians often speak of reconciliation in connection with the gospel message because that's exactly what Jesus accomplished through His death and resurrection. Our world was broken because of sin, and we as human beings were separated from God because of our rebellion against Him.

But when Jesus sacrificed Himself on the cross, He paved the way for our broken world to be restored—for the damage caused by sin to be repaired. In the same way, He gave all people a chance to become reconnected with God through His forgiveness of our sin. That's reconciliation.

Here's how Paul summarized this idea:

> In [Christ] all the fullness of God was pleased to dwell, and
> through him to reconcile to himself all things, whether on earth
> or in heaven, making peace by the blood of his cross.
> **COLOSSIANS 1:19-20**

**In your own words, what does it mean that Jesus reconciled "all things"
(v. 20) to Himself?**

Maybe you're wondering, *What does all this have to do with work?* The work we do
is part of the "all things" mentioned in verse 20. In other words, Jesus' sacrifice
paved the way for our work to be reconciled to God just like everything else.

The gospel of Jesus Christ and the message of His cross can bring purpose, value,
and joy back to a man's work. Because of the gospel you're no longer forced to
work in vain. Because of the cross you no longer have to chase the wind. Thanks
to the reconciliation Christ provided, our work can be infused with meaning and
even joy.

But it doesn't just happen. We have to actively move toward and accept the redemp-
tion we've been offered in our work. So let's consider three big steps we can take
to infuse joy and purpose into the work God has given us:

1. Embrace your current work.

2. "Work heartily, as for the Lord" (Col. 3:23).

3. Focus on the eternal value of your work.

EMBRACE YOUR CURRENT WORK

It's true that lots of people don't enjoy their jobs, but here's something to keep in
mind: whatever work you do right now is God's will for you in this moment. Your
current work is part of God's plan. So embrace it.

Acts 17:26 helps us understand this idea:

> He made from one man every nation of mankind to live
> on all the face of the earth, having determined allotted
> periods and the boundaries of their dwelling place.

Yes, God may eventually call you to do something different with your life, but right now He's calling you to do what you're doing right now. Find peace in that. And don't be afraid to ask God to give you a sense of contentment in what you're doing.

What that basically means is that you don't work for your boss—not ultimately. Instead, you work for God.

"WORK HEARTILY, AS FOR THE LORD"

Here's a question worth considering. Who's your boss? Most of us have an immediate supervisor of some sort who's responsible for overseeing and, hopefully, supporting our work. So who's yours?

Whom would you identify as your immediate supervisor?

What emotions do you experience when you think about your immediate supervisor? Why?

Just as it's true that many people don't like the work they currently do, many people also feel distaste for the bosses, supervisors, and managers who oversee that work. If that's the case in your situation, here's some good news from the Book of Colossians:

> Whatever you do, work heartily, as for the Lord and not for men,
> knowing that from the Lord you will receive the inheritance
> as your reward. You are serving the Lord Christ.
> **COLOSSIANS 3:23-24**

That phrase "as for the Lord and not for men" (v. 23) is vitally important for any man who's seeking to find joy and purpose in his work. That's because it reminds us that God is in charge of this universe.

As the Creator and Sustainer of all things, God is aware of everything that's going on in your life, including your struggles at work. He sees what you're dealing with. He sees the obstacles in front of you and the frustration you experience dealing with the same problems day after day. But through it all He's reminding you to trust Him and serve Him, even at work.

Given that God is our ultimate Boss, we can't lose sight of that first phrase from Colossians 3:23: "Whatever you do, work heartily."

It doesn't matter whether you're the CEO of a Fortune 500 company or the low man in an organization making paperclips; God invites you to work heartily for Him. That means, when it comes to your job, you're called to give everything you've got. Why? Because you're using work as an opportunity to serve God and demonstrate trust in Him, not simply to make paperclips, fix plumbing, teach children, manage call screeners, or do anything else at work.

Let's be honest: we've all been tempted to give less than 100 percent in our jobs. We're tempted to tap the brakes when nobody else is looking or maybe to figure out the minimum we need to do in order to get by and meet the expectations placed on us, especially when we don't feel that our extra efforts are appreciated or even noticed.

When are you tempted to give less than 100 percent at work?

All that changes when we focus on God as our ultimate Boss, because every day at work becomes a new opportunity to achieve authentic success by trusting Him and serving Him. We don't need earthly rewards or attention, because we under-stand that God sees and has promised us an inheritance as our reward (see v. 24).

Remember, "You are serving the Lord Christ" (v. 24). Next we'll explore another step for claiming Jesus' reconciliation in our jobs: focusing on the eternal value of our work.

WORK AND YOU

COLT'S STORY

People usually see professional football players only on game days, typically on Sundays. But have you ever wondered what guys like me do the rest of the time? Here's a quick look at my typical workweek.

During the regular season we practice on Monday. That typically involves watching film of our most recent game, both as a team and in our individual-position groups. We want to see what we did well and how we can improve.

Tuesday is our day off—our "weekend," for lack of a better word. Even so, a few players show up for a couple of hours on Tuesdays. I'm one of them. As a quarterback, I often go in on Tuesdays for a good portion of the day to get a head start on the week because I need to know what our game plan is going to be.

Every player on the team is expected to show up the rest of the week. We practice Wednesday through Friday, and those days include more film study, classroom time, and work on the field. Saturday is travel day when we have away games, but we still do a walk-through for our game plan before getting on the plane. Sunday is game day, of course, and then it starts all over again.

The average practice looks different, depending on whether you play offense or defense. Because I'm a quarterback, my day is full every day. I get to the facility about 6:00 a.m., have breakfast, look over what we're going to do for the day, then watch film, either of our previous day's practice or of our upcoming opponent. We have our regular team meeting at 9:00 a.m. Then we divide up and go into specific meetings for either offense or defense. I meet with the offensive line, the receivers, and the running backs. Then we go through a walk-through of the next set of drills and plays at 11:00 a.m.

At noon we have lunch. Right after lunch everybody gets taped up, and we all go to the field for practice. Usually we practice for 1½ to 2 hours, then come back inside for more meetings. As we watch the day's practice on film, we talk about corrections we need to make in preparation for Sunday. Right after the debriefing is finished, I go to the weight room, or if I'm injured, I go to the training room for treatment.

On most days I go home around 6:00 p.m. For me, work means a long day every day. I'm not just a guy who walks out onto the field on Sunday, plays a game, then does nothing the rest of the week. I have to work just like you, and it's tough. It can even be a grind.

Thankfully, I had good teachers at home and at church who encouraged me early on to "work heartily, as for the Lord and not for men." In fact, Colossians 3:23 has been my favorite verse for years. I still have bad days, of course. I still get frustrated and disappointed when things don't go my way or when I run up against tough situations.

But eventually, I always come back to the fact that God is my ultimate Boss, and I work for Him in everything I do.

Describe some of the best parts of your current workweek.

What parts of your workweek are more frustrating or difficult to handle?

What kind of work do you hope to be doing in five years? Why?

FOCUS ON THE ETERNAL VALUE OF YOUR WORK

Earlier we looked at the importance of focusing on God as our ultimate Boss. Whatever work we find ourselves doing, we need to "work heartily, as for the Lord and not for men" (Col. 3:23).

In the same way, it's also important for us to focus on our opportunities to do something of eternal value with our work. Yes, we can give 100 percent of our effort while fixing a pipe or writing a contract, because we know God is our true Boss. But that doesn't mean those things will make a real difference in our lives or in the lives of others. It doesn't mean those tasks will scratch our itch to do something meaningful.

But what would happen if a plumber intentionally engaged his customers in meaningful conversations whenever possible, including conversations about the gospel? What if a manager insisted on honesty in all of his contracts because he wants to be a positive witness for Jesus? These things have eternal value. They have the potential to matter not just for weeks or months but literally for eternity.

When have you seen ordinary activities result in spiritual fruit?

Who among your friends and family members is good at finding eternal value in the normal circumstances of life and work?

It's certainly true that some types of work provide more obvious opportunities for eternal value than others. For example, working as a pastor provides more chances for spiritual fruit on the surface than working as an NFL quarterback. Does that mean all quarterbacks should throw down their pads and go to seminary instead? Certainly not. God can use quarterbacks to produce fruit in the same way He uses pastors.

What it means is that quarterbacks need to spend a little extra energy identifying opportunities to seek eternal value in their jobs. The same is true for plumbers, managers, teachers, carpenters, contractors, mechanics, editors, and so on.

Do you see a lot of opportunities for spiritual fruit in your current work? Explain.

Ephesians 4:28 is a surprising passage that helps us understand this idea:

Let the thief no longer steal, but rather let him labor,
doing honest work with his own hands, so that he may
have something to share with anyone in need.

Did you catch how radical that is? This verse instructs a thief to quit his thieving ways and work instead. That's not surprising, but the verse doesn't stop there. The thief is told to go forward and, instead of stealing, do something eternally significant with his time, energy, and talents. Instead of stealing, he's supposed to work so that he can share with those who are in need.

If that's the high standard a thief is held to, how much greater is that standard for you and me? Here's the question you need to ask yourself, no matter what kind of work you currently do: *What can I do through this job that will be eternally significant?* In other words: *How can I use this job in which God has placed me to make an eternal difference?*

Record three answers to the previous questions.
1.

2.

3.

Finding eternal significance in your work might require a bit of discovery as you pray about it before the Lord and trust Him with the work He's entrusted to you. Remember, trusting God is a vital part of achieving authentic success in your life.

Work is a good thing, even though it's been corrupted by sin. Work is what we're supposed to do with much of our time in this life. We hope you'll work hard and use all of your God-given talents to achieve your goals. We hope you'll find a specific calling in life that complements your general calling to follow Jesus.

Most of all, though, we hope you're embracing the work you're doing now. We hope you're serving the Lord and not your earthly boss. We hope you're looking for ways to make an eternal impact through the tasks you've been called to do—even today. Those three truths add up to a real win in this life.

1. Andre Agassi, *Open: An Autobiography* (New York: Knopf, 2009), 3.

WEEK 5.
PURSUIT

WELCOME BACK
TO THIS GROUP DISCUSSION OF *THE REAL WIN.*

The previous session's application activity challenged you to glorify God by praying to Him during the least enjoyable portions of your work. How did it go?

Describe what you liked best about the study material in week 4. What questions do you have?

ACTIVITY. As a group, use the following questions to explore and evaluate the intersection of men and romantic love in today's culture.

- Who among your friends and family does a good job of modeling romantic love as a husband, fiancé, or boyfriend?

- As a group, identify some common elements among these men. (Consider recording these elements on a whiteboard or on a large sheet of paper.)

- Whom does our culture lift up as an ideal version of a romantic man? (Think movies, TV shows, books, and so on.)

- What are the similarities and differences between the real men we've talked about and the ideal version of romantic men from our culture?

To prepare to watch the DVD segment, read aloud the following verses.

> Husbands, love your wives, as Christ loved the church and gave himself up for her, that he might sanctify her, having cleansed her by the washing of water with the word, so that he might present the church to himself in splendor, without spot or wrinkle or any such thing, that she might be holy and without blemish. In the same way husbands should love their wives as their own bodies. He who loves his wife loves himself.
> **EPHESIANS 5:25-28**

WATCH DVD session 5.

DISCUSS the DVD segment with your group, using the following questions.

What did you like best about the visual elements in the DVD segment?

What did you like best about the discussion between Colt and Matt? Why?

Describe some of the qualities necessary to be a good husband in today's world.

Whether you're married or single, how have you fallen short of those qualities?

Matt said this about his marriage: "God gave me a second chance. ... I missed; I completely missed the mark. But God gave me another shot." What would it look like for you to have a second chance as a husband or boyfriend?

What are your goals as a boyfriend or husband in the next year? The next 10 years?

How can we as a group help and support one another as we pursue those goals?

APPLICATION. Think about some of the main activities or hobbies to which you give your passion and pursuit each week—work, sports, food, music, TV, hobbies, friends, school, and so on. Commit to give up one or two of these activities in the coming week in order to focus on pursuing the woman who matters most. If you are single, focus your attention on your girlfriend or on someone in your life who is important to you.

THIS WEEK'S SCRIPTURE MEMORY. Ephesians 5:25:

> Husbands, love your wives, as Christ loved the
> church and gave himself up for her.

ASSIGNMENT. Read week 5 and complete the activities before the next group experience.

Moving **Closer**

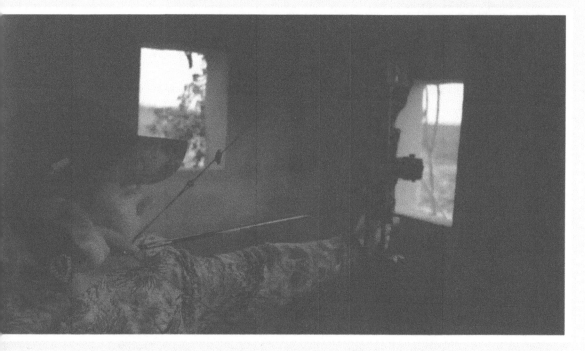

If you've ever hunted a deer, you know there are basically two options when it comes to your choice of weapons: a gun or a bow. The overall experience of the hunt is similar with both weapons; you still have to prepare in advance, know your location, and make a good shot when an opportunity presents itself.

But there's one major difference between hunting with a gun and hunting with a bow: distance. With a decent long-range rifle it's reasonable to shoot a deer at a range of 200 yards or more, sometimes even 300 yards. That means you can set up a tree stand at the edge of a cornfield or another wide-open space where there's deer traffic and just wait. If you see a target as many as two or three football fields away, you can still make the shot and harvest the animal.

Bow hunting is much more intimate. The maximum range for a kill shot with most modern bows is 50 yards, and that's pushing it. To have a reasonable chance at a successful hunt, you probably need to keep your shot to under 30 yards—not even 100 feet.

In other words, bow hunting requires a much closer pursuit of the deer. It forces you to be more intentional and more deliberate in your approach. You have to know the animal's needs and habits in order to get close enough for a successful shot.

As we'll see this week, distance is also an important principle when it comes to a man's relationship with his wife. Any husband can keep his wife at arm's length and wait for a chance to show some romance every now and again—flowers on Valentine's Day, jewelry on the anniversary, and sex whenever possible.

But the best husband—the husband who understands what the real win looks like in a marriage—makes an effort to intentionally and consistently pursue the heart of his wife.

WIN YOUR MARRIAGE

MATT'S STORY

Here's something you might not hear every day: one of the most important turning points in my marriage was sparked by my wife's encounter with another man. I'll get to that story in a minute, but first some background.

I've been married for 16 years as of the writing of this study, and I was a miserable failure as a husband for the first 10, so much so that my wife became despondent because of our relationship. And you know what's really pathetic? I had no idea anything was wrong.

During the first decade of our life together, Jennifer and I almost never argued. My wife is a laid-back person who doesn't complain. She loves and follows Jesus. So in many ways she was doing fine without my leading her or engaging with her as I should have. Meanwhile, I went happily along thinking everything was all right.

To be honest, I felt our marriage was smooth because I was a rock-star husband. I thought I had everything figured out.

Then one day my wife sat down with me to talk, but before she could get any words out, she broke down in tears. When she was finally able to speak, she said, "Matt, I want you to understand that I'd never leave you or cheat on you. But our marriage just isn't working right now."

I was shocked. "What do you mean, Jenn? What's going on?" Remember, I thought I was one of the best husbands around.

"Even when you're here, Matt, you're just not *here*," she said. "We're distant, and I never feel connected to you. When we were dating, you totally pursued me. But when we got married, you stopped pursuing me." Then she got to the heart of her feelings: "You pursue the church. You pursue your work. But you don't pursue *me*."

I was still trying to get my mind around what she was saying, so I asked for an example. Jenn was quiet for a long time. Then she told me something that had happened on a recent Sunday morning after church.

It had already been a full morning, and she was walking out to our car with our three young children in tow, plus a stroller, a diaper bag, and all the other stuff young moms need to cart around when they have little kids. I was off somewhere else, as usual, busy with church stuff, but a well-meaning man saw she was struggling to juggle everything and offered to help. He opened her car door and helped corral our kids into the backseat.

This guy did everything a good husband should have done in that situation. Nothing more happened. The guy said, "Have a good day" and walked away.

"I'd never ever cheat on you," Jenn repeated as she told me the story, "but I want you to know how good it felt for a man to pay attention to me."

At that moment I realized for the first time how poor a husband I'd been. I'd emotionally neglected my wife to the point that a simple act of kindness from a random man filled an empty place in her heart. Our conversation woke me up in a big way, and I realized there's a lot more to being a good husband than I'd considered.

What did your father teach you about being a good husband?

What have you learned from the church about being a good husband?

WHAT WOMEN NEED

You can hardly turn on the TV without encountering an exaggerated example of husbands in today's culture. These men are usually exaggerated in one of two directions: they're either total buffoons or perfect gentlemen.

The total-buffoon husbands are the guys who do the right thing only by accident. These guys are typically overweight, have foul mouths, and don't care about anybody or anything except how to get their hands on the next can of beer. Homer Simpson is a good example of a total-buffoon husband.

On the other end of the spectrum, some husbands portrayed in movies and TV shows are perfect gentlemen. These guys look good, dress well, and know how to pour on the charm. They say the right things and know how to make the women around them feel special. Coach Taylor from "Friday Night Lights" is a good example of a perfect-gentleman husband.

What can we learn from the way husbands are represented in today's culture? Obviously, we want to avoid acting like the buffoonish guys who think only about themselves and provoke contempt in the minds of their wives and families.

But we can also glean information from the behavior of those perfect-gentlemen husbands. Specifically, it's interesting that the men portrayed most positively in our culture are the ones who are intentional about pursuing the women they care about. These men go to great lengths to prove their love—and not just in the big things. They also do little things every day to make their women feel cherished, adored, and appreciated.

There's a deep need in the soul of every woman—whether it's your girlfriend, fiancée, wife, or daughter—to be cherished, pursued, and loved by the man God has placed in her life. Notice this is a *need,* not a want. If you're married (or if you'd like to be), your wife was created with a need to be pursued and cherished. She can't be herself if that need is unmet, and it's your responsibility to meet it.

> How have you seen the women in your life display the need to be cherished and pursued?

> Who are some men among your friends and family who do a good job of meeting that need for the women they love?

Thankfully, we don't have to depend on our culture's view of husbands to figure out what women need and how men should behave. The Bible has a lot to say about husbands and wives. Look at Song of Solomon, for example. The entire book is dedicated to the celebration of romantic love, and the husband involved makes a point to actively pursue his bride and make her feel cherished above all others. Look at some of his words:

Behold, you are beautiful, my love,
behold, you are beautiful!
Your eyes are doves
behind your veil.
Your hair is like a flock of goats
leaping down the slopes of Gilead.
Your teeth are like a flock of shorn ewes
that have come up from the washing,
all of which bear twins,
and not one among them has lost its young.
Your lips are like a scarlet thread,
and your mouth is lovely.
Your cheeks are like halves of a pomegranate
behind your veil.
SONG OF SOLOMON 4:1-3

What's your initial reaction to this passage? Why?

What's the most romantic thing you've ever said to your wife?
How did she respond?

Talk about pursuit! But that's not all the Scriptures teach husbands. Colossians 3:19 says, "Husbands, love your wives, and do not be harsh with them." You should treat your wife gently, with care and respect.

Peter wrote:

Husbands, live with your wives in an understanding
way, showing honor to the woman as the weaker vessel,
since they are heirs with you of the grace of life.
1 PETER 3:7

You're to actively honor your wife and make her feel special; you're commanded to be understanding. But the key passage for men and husbands is Ephesians 5:25. That's what we'll focus on when you're ready to continue your study.

LOVE YOUR WIFE

What does it look like when a husband loves his wife? That's the big question we'll explore in the next few pages. The following words from Ray Ortlund can help us wrap our brains around the issues involved:

> In the heart of every fallen woman is the self-doubt that wonders, "Do I please you? Am I what you wanted?" A wise husband will understand that question at the center of his wife's heart. And he will spend his life answering it, communicating to her in various ways, "Darling, you are the one I need. I cherish you."[1]

That's what we mean when we talk about loving your wife.

What emotions do you experience when you read the previous quotation? Why?

How have you answered the question at the center of your wife's heart?

The Bible gives you clear advice on how to actively, intentionally answer that question for your wife. You'll find it here:

> The husband is the head of the wife even as Christ is the head of the church, his body, and is himself its Savior. Now as the church submits to Christ, so also wives should submit in everything to their husbands. Husbands, love your wives, as Christ loved the church and gave himself up for her, that he might sanctify her, having cleansed her by the washing of water with the word, so that he might present the church to himself in splendor, without spot or wrinkle or any such thing, that she might be holy and without blemish. In the same way husbands should love their wives as their own bodies. He who loves his wife loves himself.
> **EPHESIANS 5:23-28**

96

What's your initial reaction to these verses?

What do you think it means to love your wife as Christ loved the church?

A lot is contained in that Scripture passage, but let's focus on verse 25: "Husbands, love your wives, as Christ loved the church and gave himself up for her."

HUSBANDS, LOVE

Notice how the first two words of Ephesians 5:25 form a short, simple, and powerful command: "Husbands, love." That's really what the pursuit is all about. If you're a husband, you're called to love the woman who gave you that title.

Also notice that it's an active command. You have to *do* something in order to love. You can't demonstrate your love by doing nothing.

What actions do you typically take when you want to show your wife that you love her?

How does your wife typically receive those actions?

When we keep reading Ephesians 5:25, we see "Husbands, love your wives, *as Christ loved the church*" (emphasis added). That's another important point. You need to love your wife in the same way Jesus loved the church.

One of the most important things we need to realize is that Jesus loved the church *first*. He initiated the love relationship between Himself and the church. In other words, Jesus didn't sit back with His arms folded and expect us as Christians to approach Him, love Him, serve Him, and then hope He'd love us back.

No, in spite of our dysfunctions, shortcomings, failures, and sins, Jesus initiated a relationship with us. He loved us first. He loved us in spite of everything. That's why 1 John 4:19 says, "We love because he first loved us."

Let's be honest and admit we don't naturally think this way in our relationships with other people, especially in our marriages. We expect to be loved first, and then we're willing to reciprocate with our own demonstrations of love. As a husband, maybe you expect to receive respect and admiration from your wife. You expect to have your needs taken care of and your desires satisfied, and then you'll show your love in return. But that's not how Christ loved the church, and that's not how you're called to pursue and cherish your wife: "Husbands, love your wives, as Christ loved the church."

> On a scale of 1 to 10, how likely are you to take the initiative when showing love to your wife?
>
> 1   2   3   4   5   6   7   8   9   10
> Not likely   Very likely

When you consider specific actions you can take to pursue and cherish your wife, it's best to start by understanding the ways she prefers to receive love. You may have heard about a book called *The Five Love Languages* by Gary Chapman. Its premise is that everybody receives love in at least one of five different ways.

- **Acts of service.** You say, "Let me do that for you." It can be anything from vacuuming the stairs to doing the dishes.

- **Gifts.** Use thoughtful gestures to demonstrate love. Bring your wife a bouquet of flowers after work, for example, or take her shopping for new clothes.

- **Physical touch.** Hugs, holding hands, and other forms of physical affection demonstrate love.

- **Words of affirmation.** You show love by speaking words of encouragement and approval: "I really care for you." "I love you deeply." "You're doing a great job."

- **Quality time.** You demonstrate love by actively listening to your spouse, which means giving your full, undivided attention for long periods of time. This can include conversations over coffee, long walks on the beach, and so on.[2]

What's your primary love language—the way you like to be loved?

How does your wife demonstrate her love for you by using that language?

What is your wife's primary love language?

How can you demonstrate love to your wife through her primary love language?

Maybe you've run into problems because you've reversed the order and tried to show love for your wife by using *your own* love language. You understand what makes you feel loved—physical touch is usually a big one for guys—so you try to express your love to your wife the same way.

That's backward. If you want to pursue and cherish your wife, you need to actively and intentionally love her in the ways she prefers to receive your love.

GIVE YOURSELF

Let's finish up the instruction from Ephesians 5:25: "Husbands, love your wives, as Christ loved the church *and gave himself up for her*" (emphasis added).

As the Head of the church, Jesus could have exercised His authority in any way He wanted. But how did He lead the church? By giving Himself up for it. And in Jesus' case, specifically, He laid His life down to show love for His people and initiate a relationship with us.

When have you been in a situation that called you to put your wife's needs above your own? What happened?

You've probably never been put in a place where you needed to die for your wife. But there are a lot of other ways you can give yourself up for the woman you love.

Think about personal purity, for example. As a man, you're called to be faithful to your wife in both mind and deed; you've promised to receive sexual pleasure and satisfaction from her and no one else. You want your wife to feel secure and confident in your commitment to her alone.

Therefore, you have several opportunities to sacrifice your personal freedom and flexibility for the sake of your wife. You can refuse to travel alone or stay in a hotel by yourself, for example. You can make sure your phone, tablet, and personal computer are protected by software that blocks inappropriate content. You can commit to the same bedtime as your wife so that you don't face temptation alone. You can give your wife open access to your texts, emails, and social media.

How would you be affected if you adopted the previous precautions for personal purity?

How would adopting the previous measures for personal purity affect your relationship with your wife?

Another way you can give yourself up for your wife is in the area of conflict. When you disagree with your wife, you might feel a strong pull to "win" the resulting argument—to come out ahead and get your own way.

But you'll approach conflict in a completely different way if your goal is to love and cherish your wife—to sacrifice yourself for her benefit—instead of to win an argument and look good in front of your buddies.

What steps can you take to put your wife first during a conflict?

Remember that authentic success comes in this life when you trust God and serve Him. That's the real win. One of the greatest opportunities you've been given to experience that win is to trust God enough to accept His guidance for pursuing and cherishing your wife and then to serve Him by serving the woman you love.

LEAD YOUR WIFE

COLT'S STORY

I've been married since 2010, and I love my wife more than I ever thought possible. We're at a really good place in our marriage now, but it hasn't always been that way. Honestly, there have been some times when I just plain blew it as a husband.

The rockiest of those times sprang from my heavy work schedule and other job challenges. Frankly, it's been hard for me to love my wife as Christ loved the church and to serve her first when my entire world revolves around football. I've known since my first day as a husband that I'm supposed to make a priority of loving and serving my wife, but I haven't always known how best to go about it.

For example, Rachel and I went through a rough patch in relation to my behavior whenever I came home from work. During our first year together I'd arrive home from the practice facility and plop down on the couch, ready for some alone time. I was ready for dinner when I got home, but I kept telling myself I didn't have the energy to engage with my wife or interact with her after a hard day.

Things finally got to the point where Rachel asked to sit down with me and have a talk. Her personality is supersweet, but she still made it clear that I wasn't living up to the expectations she had for me as a husband. "With the amount of time you spend on football," she said, "it's like I don't even have a husband."

That hurt.

I've since learned that quality time is one of my wife's main love languages. So today I make a greater effort to spend time with her and talk with her intentionally. I ask, "How are you doing? How was your day? What went on today? Whom have you talked to? How's your family? How's my family? How's your walk with Jesus?" Our conversations together have become much more meaningful. I know she appreciates the change, and so do I.

A more difficult example of my struggles as a husband has been the area of prayer. Now I pray a lot. I pray before I go to bed, at meals, and during my quiet times with the Lord. I even pray sometimes in the middle of games. But for some reason I struggled to pray with my wife early in our marriage.

As a new husband, I knew I was supposed to pray with my wife. I'd read and heard in sermons for years that praying as a married couple is essential, but when we sat down together to eat or lay down together at night, for some reason I just couldn't bring myself to say the words. Basically, I was aware of what I needed to do, but I lacked the courage and the know-how to make it happen.

These days my marriage is at a better place both relationally and spiritually. But I don't think my struggles as a husband are unique. In fact, I think most men could use a little instruction on how to be the husbands God wants us to be. It's not that marriage is a huge burden or that our wives are unlovable. It's just that we need guidance on how best to love and cherish our wives in a way that meets their needs and answers the secret questions in their hearts.

So let's finish this week by exploring what it means to love your wife as you fulfill your role as the spiritual leader in your home.

When have you worked to overcome a difficult situation in your marriage?

What are some areas in which you still have room for improvement as a husband?

What ideas or images come to mind when you hear the phrase *spiritual leader?*

SPIRITUAL LEADERSHIP

We're finishing our fifth week looking at the real win—the idea that we experience authentic success in life by trusting God and committing to serve Him. This week we've seen how being a great husband involves actively loving your wife and pursuing her heart day after day. But how do those ideas connect to the real win? What does loving and cherishing your wife have to do with authentic success?

There are two ways to answer that question, and the first is pretty basic: God has commanded you through His Word to love your wife "as Christ loved the church and gave himself up for her" (Eph. 5:25); therefore, you obey God's command when you love and cherish the woman He's placed in your care.

The second way to answer that question is to recognize that the best gift you can give your wife is to help her experience authentic success for herself—to do whatever you can to bring the real win to your wife.

For that reason God has called you as a husband to be the spiritual leader in your home. It's your responsibility to support, encourage, and lead your wife and children as they seek to trust God and serve Him with you. That's what it means to be a spiritual leader in the home.

> **Who are some men you know who do a great job of serving as the spiritual leaders in their homes?**

> **On a scale of 1 to 10, how confident do you feel about taking on the role of spiritual leader in your home?**
>
> 1   2   3   4   5   6   7   8   9   10
> Not confident   Very confident

Let's begin our exploration of spiritual leadership by taking a deeper look at these verses from Ephesians 5:

> Wives, submit to your own husbands, as to the Lord. For the husband
> is the head of the wife even as Christ is the head of the church, his
> body, and is himself its Savior. Now as the church submits to Christ,
> so also wives should submit in everything to their husbands.
> **EPHESIANS 5:22-24**

What's your initial reaction to these verses?

What do these verses teach about your role as a husband?

As you let these verses sink it, resist the urge to shout, "Oh, yeah!" Paul didn't write these words to make men bosses over their wives who force them to obey.

Remember in week 2 we learned that a man's role as a leader within his spheres of influence, including the home, is an assertion of responsibility rather than control. Just as Adam was held responsible for the actions of his family, men today bear responsibility for the actions of our families. We are the leaders.

This idea is further developed in Ephesians 5:25-27:

> Husbands, love your wives, as Christ loved the church and gave
> himself up for her, that he might sanctify her, having cleansed her
> by the washing of water with the word, so that he might present
> the church to himself in splendor, without spot or wrinkle or
> any such thing, that she might be holy and without blemish.

What do these verses teach about your role as a husband?

We've already discussed the idea of loving your wife as Christ loved the church, but these verses get more complicated. What do they mean, and what do they have to do with your wife?

Understand that "the washing of water" (v. 26) isn't talking about baptism. Rather, it refers to an ancient bridal practice. When this passage was written, the women in a bridal party would wash a bride-to-be with water before she was married. This ritual was primarily symbolic. It meant the bride was ready to be presented to her groom. She was clean, pure, and spotless in his sight.

As a husband, you're called to do the same thing as the spiritual leader in your home. You have a responsibility to ensure and support the purity of your wife— morally, spiritually, mentally, and emotionally. This doesn't happen with actual water, of course, but with "the word" (v. 26). In other words, you don't seek to purify your wife with your own ideas and opinions. Rather, you ensure and nurture her purity by exposing her to the truths revealed by God in the Bible.

What's your response to the previous statements? Why?

The implication is that you're washing yourself too. You're not commanded to wash your wife because you're superclean to begin with and your wife is morally dirty. As a spiritual leader, you're called to live a sanctified life first; you're called to bathe yourself daily in the cleansing water of God's Word. Then, instead of viewing your wife or girlfriend as someone you use for your own selfish gain, you're to lead her down the same path of sanctification you're already traveling.

That's your call: to actively support your spouse as she learns to trust and serve God so that she'll be ready to be presented "holy and without blemish" (v. 27) to her ultimate Bridegroom, Jesus Christ.

So how are you doing as a spiritual leader in your home? Take a look at the following chart and evaluate your spiritual leadership.

Do you regularly lead your wife in prayer?	YES	NO
Have you led your family to be active members of a local church?	YES	NO
Do you understand your wife's spiritual gifts and the ways she uses them to minister?	YES	NO
Do you confess your sins to your wife?	YES	NO
Do you create a culture of grace that allows your wife to grow without expecting perfection?	YES	NO
Do you create opportunities for your wife to be mentored by spiritually mature women?	YES	NO
Do you encourage your wife to serve as a spiritual role model for younger women?	YES	NO

Husbands, love your wives. Husbands, lead your wives. As you seek to trust God and serve Him, encourage and support your wife to do the same. When you take these commands to heart and live them each day, it's like strapping a rocket booster onto your journey toward authentic success.

1. Ray Ortlund, "Husband and Wife," *The Gospel Coalition* [online], 13 February 2010 [cited 5 April 2013]. Available from the Internet: *http://thegospelcoalition.org*.
2. Paraphrased from Gary Chapman, *The Five Love Languages* (Chicago: Northfield Publishing, 1992).

WEEK 6.

LEGACY

WELCOME BACK
TO THIS GROUP DISCUSSION OF *THE REAL WIN.*

The previous session's application activity challenged you to give up something you typically pursue in order to focus your attention on the woman who matters most in your life. If you're comfortable, share what happened this past week.

Describe what you liked best about the study material in week 5. What questions do you have?

ACTIVITY. Define the kind of legacy you'd like to leave in this world by filling in the blanks for the sample obituary below.

_____ [your name] died Sunday due to _____. He is survived by his wife, _____; his children, _____; and many close friends. Among his achievements in life, _____ [your name] was best known for _____ and for his work in _____. His principal motto in life was _____, and he strove to live those words each day.

To prepare to watch the DVD segment, read aloud the following verses.

> Have this mind among yourselves, which is yours in Christ Jesus, who, though he was in the form of God, did not count equality with God a thing to be grasped, but made himself nothing, taking the form of a servant, being born in the likeness of men. And being found in human form, he humbled himself by becoming obedient to the point of death, even death on a cross. Therefore God has highly exalted him and bestowed on him the name that is above every name, so that at the name of Jesus every knee should bow, in heaven and on earth and under the earth, and every tongue confess that Jesus Christ is Lord, to the glory of God the Father.
> **PHILIPPIANS 2:5-11**

WATCH DVD session 6.

DISCUSS the DVD segment with your group, using the following questions.

What did you like best about the visual elements in the DVD segment?

What did you like best about the discussion between Colt and Matt? Why?

What ideas or images come to mind when you hear the word *legacy*?

Looking at your sample obituary, how would you summarize the legacy you want to leave for the friends and family members who come behind you?

How would you summarize your current legacy if you died tomorrow?

Respond to Matt's statement: "We get to be men that don't live for ourselves. We get to be men that don't live for frivolous things that aren't going to last. But we get to live, as Jesus lived, for the glory of God."

What obstacles or hindrances can prevent you from leaving the legacy you desire? What steps can you take to overcome them?

APPLICATION. During the coming week spend some time studying the life of a man you admire—a man who left a legacy of glorifying God and investing his time and energy in pursuits that have eternal value. Read a biography or watch a documentary about that man's life. As you do so, contemplate the current trajectory of your life and the legacy you'll leave behind.

THIS WEEK'S SCRIPTURE MEMORY. Matthew 5:14:

> You are the light of the world.
> A city set on a hill cannot be hidden.

ASSIGNMENT. Read week 6 and complete the activities to conclude this study.

Making Memories

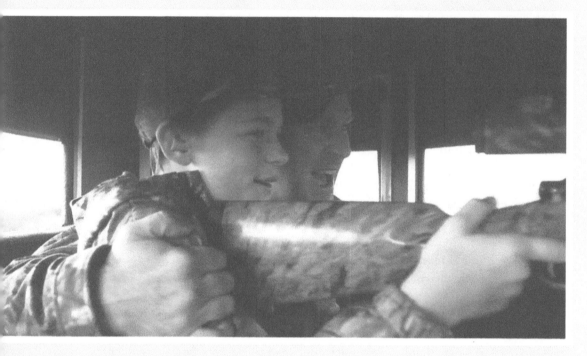

Would you agree there's something magical
about the first time we accomplish something
significant or achieve a desired goal? Think about
your first kiss, for example, or the first time you
saw the ocean. What kinds of memories do you
still carry from the first house you purchased
or the first job you landed as an adult?

A hunter may harvest dozens of animals over the course of his life, and there's no way he can remember the detailed story surrounding each kill. But he *will* remember the first time he saw an animal go down because he pulled the trigger or released his bow.

A fisherman can literally pull hundreds of fish from the water over decades spent on docks, in boats, and on the banks of rivers and lakes. He probably couldn't remember all of the different species he's caught when his fishing career is over, but he *will* remember that thrilling moment when for the first time he pulled back on his rod, set the hook, and reeled in a fish.

One reason these first times create such powerful memories is that they can't be repeated. You can never have another first catch, first kill, or first kiss.

We'll focus on this concept of memory during our final week of study, specifically in terms of the desire each of us has to be remembered for what we've accomplished. We'll also explore God's calling for each man to make an impact for eternity as we try to understand what it means to leave a legacy of authentic success.

THE BEST LEGACY

COLT'S STORY

In October 2010 the University of Texas awarded me a great and unexpected honor: it officially retired my number 12 jersey. That means no other Texas Longhorn will ever wear my number for as long as the Texas football program exists. I didn't fully understand what a big deal this was until I learned that only five other football players in the history of the University of Texas have had their jerseys retired. I'd joined a select group.

Quite frankly, the award surprised me when I first heard about it. I felt grateful and proud about what I'd been able to accomplish for my team and my school. The award also got me thinking about my legacy, both in sports and in life.

In the world of sports, the term *legacy* has pretty specific connotations. Your legacy as an athlete is all about your statistics and accomplishments on the field. These are the things fans talk about when they're trying to figure out whether someone belongs in the Pro Bowl or the Hall of Fame.

But when I think about my legacy as a person and especially as a follower of Jesus, things like having my jersey retired and whatever else I'm able to accomplish in the NFL won't be at the top of my list. Instead, I hope I'll be remembered for efforts and achievements that have eternal value.

Here's an example. When I was at the University of Texas, several guys from our football team started meeting together to study the Bible and encourage one another as followers of Christ. We didn't have a chaplain or an official leader; we just knew it was best for us to support one another in community.

In one meeting we were studying Matthew 5, and we came across this verse:

> You are the light of the world.
> A city set on a hill cannot be hidden.
> **MATTHEW 5:14**

One guy in our group said, "I've heard that term before—*COAH*. It stands for *city on a hill*. That's what I want to be like."

We asked him what he meant, and he explained that he wanted to live differently. He didn't want his identity to be based on the fact that he was a Texas football player. He wanted to be known as a person who follows Jesus.

The rest of us thought that sounded right on, so we started calling one another COAHs to remind ourselves that we had the ability to be examples and role models. Football is huge in Texas, but that wasn't the core of our identity. This title reminded us to remove any swagger that might be present in our lives. We wanted to set the standard and be the light God wanted us to be.

Pretty soon other guys started joining the study, and several of them didn't have much experience with church or the Bible. One night after practice we were meeting, and the subject of baptism came up. Lots of guys had different opinions, and a few of the new guys had no idea what we were talking about. So we dove into the Scriptures and started figuring out what it means to be baptized and why all Christians should be baptized as a public declaration of their faith. I'd been baptized when I was 14, so I was able to share my experiences with the group.

In the middle of that discussion, five guys in the group decided they wanted to be baptized—and they wanted it to happen right away! There just happened to be a pool around the corner from our practice facility, so we headed over there.

I ended up baptizing all five of those guys that night. It was an incredible experience. Obviously, it didn't happen because of anything I did or didn't do; it was the Holy Spirit working in that community of guys. They wanted to fully submit their lives to Christ and obey what the Bible commanded. I'll never forget it.

In the grand scheme of things, people might remember my football career for a few decades after I retire. Having my jersey retired by the University of Texas might keep my name in people's minds after I die, but who knows how long I'll actually be remembered? People might not even play football a hundred years from now!

But what happened at the pool that night was different because it was eternally significant. My name won't be remembered, but the consequences of baptizing five of my friends and teammates will still be felt thousands and thousands of years from now.

That's the kind of legacy I want to leave.

What are some of your most impressive accomplishments so far in life? Record three.

1.

2.

3.

How have you been eternally influenced by the efforts of other people?

What are you currently investing in that has the potential to be eternally significant?

REMEMBERED OR FORGOTTEN?

Have you ever heard of Count Ludwig von Zinzendorf? The name sounds like a vampire hunter from Transylvania, but he was actually a German church leader who lived in the mid-1700s. Zinzendorf was extremely talented and dedicated to ministry. He wrote and taught extensively; worked with orphans; established communities of faith worldwide; and wrote a large number of hymns, many of which are still sung today.

If anyone deserves to be remembered for the things they did in service to Christ, Count Ludwig von Zinzendorf should be in the conversation.

But that wasn't what Zinzendorf wanted:

> The missionary must seek nothing for himself: no seat of honour,
> no report of fame. Like the cab-horses in London, the Count said, he
> must wear blinders and be blind to every danger and to every snare
> and conceit. He must be content to suffer, to die and be forgotten.[1]

Count Zinzendorf didn't work so that people would remember his good deeds. He worked, ministered, and loved the people around him so that they'd remember Jesus. That's the kind of legacy we're talking about this week.

What ideas or images come to mind when you hear the word *legacy*?

How does our culture define a successful legacy for modern men?

Most men have a built-in desire to strive and succeed. We want to climb mountains and achieve goals. We want to perform well at whatever we do, but sometimes that desire leads us to want people to *see* us perform well; we might want people to notice, be impressed, and remember our success. In other words, it's natural for us to think of our legacy in terms of our achievements and accomplishments.

But that's not the legacy we should be shooting for as followers of Christ. Instead, we need to be faithful in pursuing authentic success—faithful in trusting God and serving Him wherever we are and in whatever we do. Who cares whether we're remembered or forgotten as long as we finish the work God gives us?

On a scale of 1 to 10, how often do you think about the way others will remember you when you're gone from this world?

1   2   3   4   5   6   7   8   9   10

Almost never   Almost daily

Jesus Himself set the pattern for this kind of selflessness when pursuing the real win. Look at these words by the apostle Paul:

> Have this mind among yourselves, which is yours in Christ Jesus, who, though he was in the form of God, did not count equality with God a thing to be grasped, but made himself nothing, taking the form of a servant, being born in the likeness of men. And being found in human form, he humbled himself by becoming obedient to the point of death, even death on a cross. Therefore God has highly exalted him and bestowed on him the name that is above every name, so that at the name of Jesus every knee should bow, in heaven and on earth and under the earth, and every tongue confess that Jesus Christ is Lord, to the glory of God the Father.
> **PHILIPPIANS 2:5-11**

What strikes you as most interesting about this passage? Why?

How did Jesus demonstrate humility and selflessness in His life?

When Jesus died on the cross, it didn't look like He'd left much of a legacy. He'd written no books and accumulated no wealth. The authorities had trashed His reputation. The crowds had disappeared, and His remaining followers scattered and were ready to return to what they'd been doing before they met Jesus.

But Jesus was faithful in the redemptive work He'd been called to do. And through that faithfulness He changed the world—forever.

Don't miss verse 5 in that passage, which says we're supposed to have the same mind as Jesus—the same determination to be selflessly faithful to God and His plans. That's what a true legacy looks like.

It's not about our being remembered or our names being passed through history. Instead, the best legacy we can leave behind is to be faithful to our calling, serve God selflessly, and trust that He will take care of everything else.

DEFINE YOUR LEGACY

If you've spent time studying the Bible, you've noticed that it often conflicts with the values and principles typically held by the culture around us.

For example, today's culture tells us that life is all about living life to the fullest, having the most fun possible, and making the most of each day. But the Bible calls us to deny ourselves (see Matt. 16:24). Today's culture tells us that money and possessions are the keys to happiness, and the more we have, the better our lives will be. The Bible, however, teaches that the love of money is the root of all kinds of evil (see 1 Tim. 6:10) and that we shouldn't love the things of this world (see 1 John 2:15).

> What are some other areas in which the Bible conflicts with the values of modern society?

The same thing happens when we think about legacy. Society tells us that people are remembered and valued for their accomplishments and the impressive goals they achieve—that the ultimate goal is to achieve greatness and be remembered for generations.

But as we saw earlier, a biblical view of legacy means being faithful to God's calling. It means embracing being forgotten so that Christ can be remembered.

John Piper does a good job of summing up the Bible's perspective on legacy:

> God created us to live with a single passion: to joyfully display
> his supreme excellence in all the spheres of life. The wasted
> life is the life without this passion. God calls us to pray and
> think and dream and plan and work not to be made much
> of, but to make much of him in every part of our lives.[2]

> Whom do you know who demonstrates a genuine passion for God?

How would you describe our culture's view of a wasted life?

If we agree that achieving a legacy of authentic success means remaining faithful to our calling, we have to ask, How do we know our calling? How do we figure out the work we're supposed to do in order to glorify Christ?

We'll focus on your specific calling as an individual later. First let's explore two broad callings that apply to every man, including you.

BE A CITY ON A HILL

One way we leave a legacy that glorifies Christ is by living as a city on a hill in this world. Again, that idea comes from Jesus' teaching in Matthew 5:

> You are the light of the world. A city set on a hill cannot be hidden. Nor do people light a lamp and put it under a basket, but on a stand, and it gives light to all in the house. In the same way, let your light shine before others, so that they may see your good works and give glory to your Father who is in heaven.
> **MATTHEW 5:14-16**

What does it mean for Christians to be "the light of the world" (v. 14)?

How do we as Christians "let [our] light shine before others" (v. 16)?

Just because your ultimate legacy isn't to gain personal fame doesn't mean you'll never be *noticed* in this world. Quite the opposite. Christians aren't called to live hidden, solitary lives where people don't see us and don't know we follow Christ.

Instead, we're called to live in the real world with all sorts of people from all sorts of backgrounds and faith persuasions. Our call is to live in such a way that the light of Christ shines out from us. That means going into our churches and communities and doing the kind of work that makes a difference: loving the unlovable, ministering to widows and orphans, fighting evil where we find it, feeding the hungry, visiting prisoners, sharing the good news of Jesus, and so on.

> What are some problems in your community that could be helped or solved by good men who commit to good work? Record three.
> 1.
>
>
> 2.
>
>
> 3.
>
>
> How can you pitch in to work on one or more of those problems?

According to God's Word, the work we do should be so radical that we stand out from all other men the way a brightly lit city stands out against the night sky. We should be noticed as Christian men. But because our efforts focus on serving God instead of ourselves, we'll be noticed in such a way that people "see [our] good works and give glory to [our] Father who is in heaven" (v. 16).

To be a city on a hill means we reflect God's excellence and glory in every area of our lives. That's how we become "content to suffer, to die and be forgotten," as Count Zinzendorf talked about. That's how we live for the sake of Christ even as we do the hard work for His kingdom.

LEAVE A LEGACY WITH YOUR FAMILY

Any good work you do in your church and community can be undercut if you fail to do a greater work in your family. As a Christian man, you're called first and foremost to be the spiritual leader in your home.

We've already covered your responsibilities when it comes to leading your wife on a spiritual level, but the Bible also has a lot to say about what it means to be a godly father.

On that note Deuteronomy 6:4-9 may be one of the most practically important passages in God's Word. If you're a dad, pay close attention to what these verses say. If you're a future dad, let this passage become foundational for you even now:

> Hear, O Israel: The LORD our God, the LORD is one. You shall love the LORD your God with all your heart and with all your soul and with all your might. And these words that I command you today shall be on your heart. You shall teach them diligently to your children, and shall talk of them when you sit in your house, and when you walk by the way, and when you lie down, and when you rise. You shall bind them as a sign on your hand, and they shall be as frontlets between your eyes. You shall write them on the doorposts of your house and on your gates.

What do you find most interesting about these verses?

How did your home as a child compare to the standard set in these verses?

Dad, let the Word of God be on your heart. Study the Scriptures. Know the Scriptures. Make them a part of your routine each day so that they can change your life and the lives of those around you.

Dad, teach the Bible to your children. You don't need a seminary degree for this. Simply talk to your kids about what you experience when you study the Bible. Tell them what you learn, talk to them about the questions you wrestle with, and teach them the principles that help you make tough choices each day.

Do these things "when you sit in your house" (v. 7). That's the dinner table. Or have some meaningful conversations on the couch before you turn on the TV.

Also do these things "when you walk by the way" (v. 7). We spend so much time in our cars today, driving our kids here and there. Don't waste these opportunities. Don't default to headphones and built-in DVD players. Use the time to do the meaningful work of leading your family spiritually.

On a scale of 1 to 10, how confident are you when it comes to serving as the spiritual leader of your children?

1	2	3	4	5	6	7	8	9	10
Not confident									Very confident

What steps will you take this week to intentionally serve as the spiritual leader of your family?

Remember, the key to leading others toward authentic success is moving toward the real win yourself. This principle works in parenting. Your kids ought to be able to watch you and know what it means to be completely sold out as a follower of Jesus Christ.

This principle works in marriage. Do you want to have a rock-solid marriage? Be in love with Jesus and let that love flow through you and affect the way you love your wife.

This principle also works for single men. Do you want to walk in purity with the women you date? Be in love with Jesus. Follow in the pathway of His commands and let Him set you free to seek what He wants for your relationships. Find ways to have an impact on the next generation even if you don't have kids of your own.

Being a city on a hill and leaving a legacy with your family will take you a long way on the path of obedience to God. We'll finish up this week by focusing on the specific things He's called you to do in order to leave a godly legacy.

DEFINE YOUR CALLING

MATT'S STORY

For a long time I had no idea I'd become a pastor. In fact, I didn't want to be a pastor; I mostly planned on being a doctor when I grew up. That's the career path I would've chosen for myself.

As I began to mature, however, I eventually sensed that God wanted me to go into full-time vocational ministry. I don't remember exactly when I became aware of God's leading me in that direction; it was a gradual thing. I came to understand that He wanted me to be a pastor and wanted me to preach.

Even so, I didn't change my plans right away. I fought against what I knew He wanted. And honestly, the reason I resisted God's call was that I didn't want to be poor.

During the summer between my sophomore and junior years of college, things finally came to a head. I was working for a construction company in Texarkana at the time, and I drove back to Dallas every chance I got to see this girl named Jennifer, my future wife. So I had a lot of time to think that summer.

One afternoon I was driving on the freeway when I found myself praying and wrestling with God in a serious way. I knew He wanted me to surrender. I knew He wanted me to change the direction of my life, and I knew I didn't want to do it. I fought against giving up control and going where God was calling me to go.

Then this song came on the radio. It was a Christian song, and I'll admit parts of it were pretty cheesy. But in that moment God powerfully spoke to my heart through the words of that song.

One line in particular pointedly asked whether the listener would be the one to answer the call. And I knew God was asking that question of me. Directly. He wasn't going to let me waffle back and forth any longer. I had to make a choice.

That's when I finally surrendered. I pulled off the road and prayed to God right then and there, "Lord, I don't care where You want me to go or what You want me to do. I'm Yours. I'll do whatever You want."

That was the moment when I stopped fighting. God had been working on me and preparing me, and eventually He brought me to the place where I laid down my will and picked up His will, whatever may come.

> What were some of your life goals when you were a child? Record three.
> 1.
>
> 2.
>
> 3.
>
> When have you wrestled with God or resisted His will in the past? What happened?
>
>
> To what degree have you communicated with God about your current career?

LISTEN FOR HIS CALL

As we've seen, all men have a calling to be faithful in two broad categories: serving as a city on a hill and serving as the spiritual leader of their families. No matter what else happens in our lives, we're doing the right thing if we focus on those two goals.

But all men also have a calling from God—something God has uniquely designed them to do or accomplish. For example, Colt McCoy's calling is to serve as a professional quarterback, at least for the next several years. Matt Carter's calling is to serve as the pastor of a church. What about you?

> How would you describe your calling in life?

Does the current trajectory of your life and career match that specific calling? Explain.

Many men feel they aren't sure about their calling. They don't know exactly what God has gifted them to do in this life. And that's OK—for a time. It often takes time for us to learn enough about ourselves and experience enough to identify the specific work God wants us to do.

But eventually we need to make some tough decisions and take up the call to do what God wants us to do. Eventually you need to fulfill your calling.

The Bible says in several places that God gives spiritual gifts to His followers in order to equip them for work in His kingdom. Romans 12:4-8 is a good example:

> As in one body we have many members, and the members do not
> all have the same function, so we, though many, are one body in
> Christ, and individually members one of another. Having gifts that
> differ according to the grace given to us, let us use them: if prophecy,
> in proportion to our faith; if service, in our serving; the one who
> teaches, in his teaching; the one who exhorts, in his exhortation;
> the one who contributes, in generosity; the one who leads, with
> zeal; the one who does acts of mercy, with cheerfulness.

Circle all of the specific gifts listed in the previous verses. Which of your friends and family members demonstrate these gifts?

What specific gifts has God given you to serve Him and minister to others? Record three.

1.

2.

3.

Keep in mind that none of us create or force our calling in life. This is something God places on our minds and hearts. He initiates the call, and we respond.

Yet it's still possible for you to position yourself to know what God is saying to you and respond when that moment of calling comes. So even if you're not sure what God wants you to do in this moment, make sure you're working for Him. Obey His Word and focus on things that have eternal significance, and you'll be in a good place to hear Him when He's ready to give you a specific type of work.

If you're not sure about your calling in life, use the following steps to prepare yourself for God's call so that you can respond appropriately.

- **Inquire.** Begin by asking yourself, *Am I living for me, or am I living for the Lord?* If you're living for the Lord, that's awesome. If you're living for yourself, pray for transformation and take the steps God reveals to you in His Word and through prayer.

- **Surrender.** Stop wrestling with God. Get to a place where you say, "This is not about me, Lord. It's about You, and I'll do whatever You want me to do." You might not know exactly what you need to do, but you can put yourself in a position of surrender so that you're willing to do whatever God requires of you.

- **Prepare.** If you sense the Lord may be calling you in a specific direction, you might take classes in that area, read books, build up financial reserves, learn a new skill, or hone an existing skill to prepare to launch into your calling...... .
  . . .

- **Wait.** Wait actively and expectantly, with great faith. Psalm 46:10 encourages us to "cease striving and know that I am God" (NASB). Only God knows what will happen to you after that. He's writing your story even now, so you don't have to figure out your vision. God will reveal it to you. Seek His will through diligent Bible study and prayer.

- **Launch.** Put your seatbelt on. When God places a call on your heart, go. Be obedient. Be courageous. Choose to follow God fully, without reservations.

  Circle the stage that best describes your current stage in identifying your call. What are you doing in that stage to listen for God's voice and to seek His will?

Remember, the real win is built on two simple but strategic commitments: whom we trust and whom we serve. Those two decisions change everything for a man. When we wholeheartedly trust and serve God, we can be confident that He will lead us into a calling that will bring glory to Him and make an impact for eternity.

When it comes to legacy, it ultimately doesn't matter whether we're successful in the eyes of the world. It doesn't matter whether we fulfill the kinds of goals that fit on spreadsheets or lead to earthly fame. In Christ our hearts are satisfied.

THE REAL WINNER

Throughout this study we've talked about the real win—how to live our lives according to God's plan by trusting and serving Him. It should be clear by now that not only is there a real win in the way we live our lives, but there's also a Real Winner in the larger scope of things. Of course, the Real Winner is God.

In the grand scheme of history—from the garden, where Adam first set us men on our course of struggle with masculinity, to the distant future long after we've fulfilled our legacy—God is working to bring His perfect plan to completion. And we know from Scripture that Christ will ultimately conquer in all things. Heaven will come to earth, and everything will be made right. Forever.

God is the great Winner, so it's only appropriate that we use our lives to magnify His glory; it makes sense for us to cast away our limited plans and definitions of success in order to submit to His perfect plan. When we trust and serve Him, we become part of the greatest victory of all.

So go for the real win. Be faithful, be a leader, win the victory over idolatry, win at work, win at home, and win the future by leaving a legacy for God's glory. If a quarterback and a preacher from Texas can find authentic success in God, you can too. We're excited to think about all God is going to do in your life and, through you, in the lives of many more people around you.

1. A. J. Lewis, *Zinzendorf, the Ecumenical Pioneer* (London: SCM Press Ltd., 1962), 92.
2. John Piper, *Don't Waste Your Life* (Wheaton, IL: Crossway, 2003), 37.

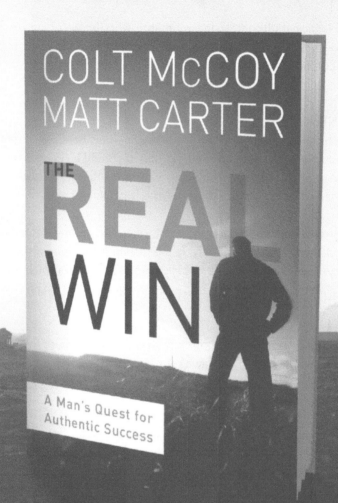
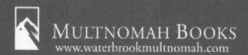